THE YOGATRONIC DIET
Amazing New Way to a Youthful, Trim Body

Other Books by Frank Rudolph Young

Secret Mental Powers: Miracle of Mind Magic

Secrets of Personal Psychic Power

Secret of Spirit-thought Magic

Somo-Psychic Power: Using Its Miracle Forces for a Fabulous New Life

Yoga For Men Only

Yoga Secrets for Extraordinary Health and Long Life

Zodic Force Control: Secret of Miracle Healing and Long Life

THE YOGATRONIC DIET
Amazing New Way to a Youthful, Trim Body

Frank Rudolph Young, D.C.

PARKER PUBLISHING COMPANY, INC.
West Nvack, NY

This book is a reference work based on research by the author. The opinions expressed herein are not necessarily those of or endorsed by the publisher. The directions stated in this book are in no way to be considered as a substitute for consultation with a duly licensed doctor.

Library of Congress Cataloging in Publication Data

Young, Frank Rudolph.
The yogatronic diet.

Includes bibliographical references and index.
1. Reducing diets. 2. Nutrition. I. Title.
RM222.2.Y68 613.2'5 79-14244
ISBN 0-13-972521-0

Printed in the United States of America

This book is dedicated to everyone who strives to look young, during early middle and late years, to everyone who seeks the way to a youthful body and a trim waist–in order to live the attractive life.

Acknowledgments

The selection in Chapter 13, from *A Text Book of Pathology: An Introduction to Medicine,* by William Boyd, M.D., is quoted by special permission from Lea & Febriger, Publishers.

The selections from "Protein Degradation: Putting the Research Together," Kolata, G. B., *Science*, Vol. 198, No. 4317, pp. 596-598. 11, November, 1977, © 1977 by the American Association for the Advancement of Science, are quoted by special permission from *Science*.

The selections from "Supression of Sympathetic Nervous System during Fasting," by Young, J. B., and Landberg, L., *Science* Vol. 196, pp. 1473-1475, 24 June 1977, © 1977 by the American Association for the Advancement of Science, are quoted by special permission from *Science* and the authors.

The 1979 Build and Blood Pressure Study of the Association of Life Insurance Medical Directors and the Society of Actuaries. Material reprinted with special permission.

Yoga for Men Only, Dr. Frank R. Young, Parker Publishing Company, Inc. West Nyack, N.Y.

what this book can do for you

You *can* become trim and youthful—and look your handsomest or most beautiful all your life, with the least effort and despite living a full, active, tense, hard life. You can do it and feel at your best, enjoy life to the utmost, function at your keenest and live healthily and long. You need not touch one stimulant, cigarette, drink, vitamin or mineral pill. You can even do it while living in polluted big cities, unavoidably consuming foods loaded with chemicals, drugs, hormones and preservatives. Indeed, you could do it without even taking more than a four day vacation four or five times in fifty years. You can do it and still feel as if *floating* in the air, bursting with ecstasy, and looking much younger than you are. I know, for *I have done it.* I did it with the *Yogatronic Diet.* So has my wife.

LONG LIFE AND THE "IDEAL WEIGHT"

Obesity is acknowledged as the leading health problem in America today. Being underweight is not desirable either; it ages your looks and shortens your life. A direct inquiry to the Metropolitan Life Insurance Company brought a prompt reply. Here, with their permission, are some quotations from it:

". . . a number of mortality investigations conducted by life insurance companies had clearly demonstrated that persons whose weight was below average lived longer than those whose weight was close to average." And, for that reason, "The primary purpose of the table of 'desirable weights' (or 'ideal weights'), developed by the Metropolitan Life Insurance Company in 1942, was to help people keep their weight down below average . . ."

The *Yogatronic Diet* enables you to achieve—in a brief time—your "ideal weight." I developed it and have had it tested on myself for over 50 years. Today, at nearly 70 years of age, I still possess the "ideal weight." My wife adopted the *Yogatronic Diet* during the 40 years of our marriage. Although inclined to gain weight easily, she also maintains her "ideal weight" year after year. Yet, we "eat like horses" and are so healthy and strong that we engage in vigorous physical activity. Mrs. Young jogs five to seven miles five days a week, while I train, with my young private disciple for four hours a day. Five nights a week, too, I climb 12 flights of stairs at top speed by 2's before going to bed.

THE YOGATRONIC DIET AND MR. UNIVERSE

Besides, I have not lost my looks with the *Yogatronic Diet*, as do so many people who follow diets. With this diet and my secret natural *Yogatronic* body movements I built myself up so symmetrically since 17 that, at 21, leading sculptors chose me to pose for their Century of Progress World's Fair statues. Hollywood scouts spotted me while modeling and chose me for stardom, without even requiring an audition. They chose me *on my physique alone*, not because I had won athletic trophies or body building awards. I had none!

At 40, with barely six weeks of two-hour-a-day intensified training, and without lifting weights or using apparatus, without taking vitamin-mineral pills or high protein concentrates to increase my muscle definition, or anabolic hormones to multiply my weight-mass, or any other body building aid, except the *Yogatronic Diet*, I competed with a host of trophy-holding body builders half my age. I was selected as a *finalist* against a famous, much-crowned body builder of 22 who trained up to eight hours a day for months, took high-protein concentrations and fistfuls of body building pills a day and won MR. AMERICA, MR. USA, MR. WORLD and MR. UNIVERSE—plus *every subdivisional* title, and retired undefeated. (You will see how I achieved it in Chapter 1). While your goals of physical appearance may be more limited, the secrets I used are for your immediate application in this easy and deeply rewarding program of health and longevity.

LIKE REVERSING THE AGING PROCESS

No matter how hard your life, no matter how full of disappointment and frustration it may be, if you stay trim and at your "ideal weight," you stay youthful. You can always make comebacks, even if you are considered too old. You will, because you will be considered far younger than you are—and be treated and sought after as if you *are* far younger. Such instant reactions of others to you will thrill you, incite you and bring out your full hidden powers: the unused 90 percent of them. The physical joy of living, your flat midsection, the exhilaration of your blood flowing easily through the unclogged blood vessels of your brain, and your looking your most handsome (or most beautiful) possible, will surpass that of a "high."

And it will be a *natural, healthy* high. It will be a high you will enjoy day after day, *without harmful side effects*. You will be energetic and youthful, and as attractive in your appearance as possible, and continue taking an active part in life!

You will look and feel more as you did when much younger. Since you are more informed and experienced than you were then, you may reach your goals much easier, faster, and more effectively.

THE PROOF OF THE PUDDING

For thirty years I have successfully taught *Yogatronics* to others, putting them on the road to a great new life. I have 24 years of accumulated evidence as to how successful and ahead of the times the *Yogatronic Diet* is. Science recently discovered the 8 Golden Rules for a long, healthy, youth-retaining happy life.[1] I myself had discovered and published these exact rules *21 years* before science revealed them. Science also recently discovered the safest, record-breaking way to reduce your weight and your waist without pills, special diet or surgery. With it, one man lost 219 lbs. in 38 weeks and reduced his waist from 50 inches to 32.[2] It turns out to be the *exact Yogatronic program* which I had already taught 25 years before, practically word-for-word. Science, though, has not yet announced finding the important 9th Golden Rule of the *Yogatronic Diet*. That rule is the Triple Tonic Secret. It is revealed in this book.

THE WONDERS OF THE YOGATRONIC DIET

1. The 8 Magic Rules promise you a long, healthy, youthful life.
2. The Triple Tonic Secret, the 9th Magic Rule, is a superhealth secret disclosed in this book.
3. Multiply the nutritive value of the devitalized food you eat, *without adding food supplements*—and it doesn't cost you a penny.
4. Neutralize the cumulative effects of the poison chemicals added to your commercial food and still be healthy, vigorous and youthful—even when you are near 70.
5. Assume the extraordinary digestive power of the gorilla and "nutrify" your tissues with less food.
6. Arouse *Power Yoga* assimilation in your body, from your skin to the innermost cells in your body, and reverse the aging process.
7. Slim down your waist in the fastest, safest *natural way*.
8. Burst with health—on supermarket foods—without adding vitamin-minerals, polyunsaturated oils, or any other food concentrate.
9. Raise your alpha-cholesterol, the wonder beneficial cholesterol, and retain your "ideal" weight.

All this *taps* the magic of the *Yogatronic Diet*—the way to eat wisely and attain the Fountain of Youth.

THE MIRACLE OF THE YOGATRONIC DIET

To my utmost satisfaction, those who followed the *Yogatronic Diet* to the letter changed their lives thoroughly—some of them in an unbelievably short time, such as a week or two. Their waistlines, their hips, their flabby arms and their shapeless torsos, all shed their unflattering bulks and acquired eye-catching contours. One after another of these excited volunteers, irrespective of age, sex or occupation, realized one dream after another which were previously pursued in long frustration. The unattractive woman suddenly fascinated man after man. The fatigued man suddenly bounded with energy. Young people and adults who were called "not too bright," suddenly bewildered others with their mental sharpness and wisdom. Several individuals whom wealth had eluded for decades, suddenly acquired the uncanny ability to make everything they touched "turn to gold." All these changes were triggered by the 9 Magic Rules of the *Yogatronic Diet.* The nutrients of the food—even of long-harvested, big city, grocery store food—"magically" infiltrated every cell of their bodies, altered its biochemistry and transformed the anatomies and physiologies of these persons, like a genie.

HOW THE YOGATRONIC DIET TRANSFORMED PEOPLE

The *Yogatronic Diet* changed both the bodies and personalities of these people. As a result, their walks changed and the looks in their eyes changed. Their sex lives, hobbies, social lives, business and professional lives, outlooks for the future, family and domestic relationships—all changed radically. Whole appearances—particularly waistlines, hips, and other malproportioned regions—changed fantastically!

Yet, to effect these incredible transformations in these people did not cost them one penny more in food. They didn't have to move to different climates. They didn't have to change their lines of work or go on fasts. Their burdensome bodies and selves were exchanged for enchanting new ones, and they had resorted to no equipment, drugs or food pills, nor had they lived on farms and raised their own foods. They had not had to compute or memorize tiresome food facts. They had bought no special clothes, nor exerted themselves additionally. Still, their lives were now totally different and brought them all the things they most desired! Look for yourself at this list of case histories of some of the many people who gained magically from the *Yogatronic Diet.* And most of them did so in from just one week to three months time.

THE UNBELIEVABLE CASE PROOF

1. Sally K. lost 20 pounds and her sallow complexion (page 63).
2. Tina U. lost her unwanted bulk and her drying up look (page 64).
3 Howard W. was soon taken for a college athlete (page 72).
4. Jesse B. doubled his company's profits in very bad times (page 72).
5. Charles F. and his wife "ate like horses," but still wore youthful clothes in their sixties (page 83).
6. Thelma Z. lost her matronly look speedily (page 83).
7. Kevin L. scaled off ugly pounds and pioneered a wealth-making enterprise (page 97).
8. Enid T. lost 30 pounds and turned irresistible (page 97).
9. The author still keeps his weight exactly constant at what it was at 20-21 (page 108).
10. Ramsey B. achieved virtual immortality (page 119).
11. Betty-Lou H. bid good-bye to her needless fat and stiffening joints (page 120).
12. Percy B. rejuvenated his mind (page 128).
13. Jane C. promptly improved every phase of her life (page 135).
14. Andrew S., through easy self-control, started a new life of exciting ventures (page 143).
15. Marcella M. sweetened her moods and transformed her husband into an overwhelming success (page 143).
16. John B. was promoted unexpectedly at retirement age (page 155).
17. Ellen K. lost 37 pounds and out-thought her rivals (page 155).
18. Louisa G. altered her image to others and was soon eagerly pursued (page 162).
19. Richard P. went from an overworked father of four to a successful actor (page 163).

20. Tom and Laura F. were transformed from the "sleepy" group to the "living" crowd (page 173).
21. Rudy V. reduced his yearly colds to a minimum (page 173).
22. Lena R. became a sylph-like tigress in her sport activity (page 184).
23. Anita Q. quickly captured a wealthy stranger for a husband (page 184).
24. Alma W., to her amusement, was suddenly offered a job as a "stripper (page 192).
25. Archie R. was unexpectedly selected for the high position he wanted (page 193).
26. Bertha A. had to start wearing long sleeves to keep the men away (page 202).
27. Hector N. trimmed down 68 pounds and felt healthier than he had since he was a youth (page 212).
38. Oona D. hung on to her handsome younger husband against much younger competition (page 212).
29. Clothilda I. catapulted herself into the beauty queen class (page 222).

One after another of these real-life testimonials could easily be duplicated by you or by somebody you wish to help. Just follow the magical, delicious way to wise eating in the *Yogatronic Diet*. In no time, you will feel as light as air and look many years younger all your life.

Frank Rudolph Young

REFERENCES

[1]School of Public Health at the University of California at Los Angeles. A 10-year study of 7,000 residents of Alameda, California.

[2]University of Mississippi.

contents

THE YOGATRONIC DIET
Amazing New Way to a Youthful, Trim Body

1

the amazing new way to a trim, youthful body

How I was Selected as a Finalist Against A Coming Mr. Universe Half My Age

At 40, I had never competed in a body-building contest and knew little about it. But when I learned that there was a *Mr. Novice* body-building contest coming up that weekend for non-trophy holders, I entered for the fun of it.

I was thoroughly beaten. Sympathizers confided to me that I knew very little about body-building posing, and that my muscles were not defined enough.

I learned about the next contest six weeks before it was to take place. The best body builders in the State would be participating in it. It would consist mainly of trophy holders who had been weight-lifting for years, many of whom held or were runners-up for national and regional titles. I determined to try the seemingly impossible and compete against them. I was sick and tired of hearing that the *Yogatronic System* did not compare in results with lifting weights or using other exercise apparatus. All the contestants, except me, belonged to gyms and had been preparing for months, putting up to four hours a day of practice for the event. I myself could afford to devote only two hours a day in the six weeks that remained, doing my natural resistance exercises at home and in the park.

But, I added something to my diet which none of them knew anything about. I "transferred" to my digestion Bushman's extraordinary digestive power. (Bushman was the late, biggest, longest lived gorilla in captivity). With that fantastic digestive power my muscles absorbed the supermarket food I ate like blotters and gained size with stupefying efficiency. They were greatly aided by the new speed-up body building discovery I made in my natural resistance program. Both, together, seemingly burned up fat faster and endowed me with amazing definition, compared to what I had before.

Despite the championship caliber of the competition I faced this time, I was selected a *finalist* with the winner. I was thunderously applauded by the crowd, a good many of whom preferred me to the winner. The winner was so incomparable, however, that he moved on to win *Mr. America*, *Mr. USA*, *Mr. World* and *Mr. Universe*, one after another, including all the subtitles, like *Best Arms*, *Best Legs*, *Best Back*, *Best Chest*, *Most Muscular*, *Best Posing*. He even scored the highest total points recorded and he retired undefeated.

For months before the national contests, though, the winner took high protein concentrates daily, fistfuls of vitamin-mineral and body building pills every two hours or so, lifted weights for a total of eight hours a day, and practiced his posing for another four hours. He trained, in brief, about 12 times more than I. For years, since then, many top body builders have even added anabolic steroids to acquire "artificially" even greater size and muscle definition. Many among the scores of top and mediocre body builders I have known personally, some of whom were rated among the top three, may have endangered their kidneys, to win by imbibing no liquids for up to three days before the contests to increase their muscular definition to the maximum. I refused to risk my health like that and did not compete again.

But I had proved to myself the miracles of the *Yogatronic Diet*. Had I, too, taken such concentrates, what a staggering "artificial" physique I would have built up! By not doing so, however, I don't have to worry about internal damage which I might have caused myself. With the *Yogatronic Diet* I have remained at my scientifically proved "ideal weight," the longevity weight. My primary goal was to find the Fountain of Youth and the secret of a healthy long life.

How Mrs. Young, My Wife, at 37, With Comparatively Little Preparation, Competed Remarkably Against Established Winners Half Her Age

When my wife was 37 she had worked for 16 years, had been married for seven, and had not competed in sports for 20. I refused to let her join the sedentary middle-aged, however, for she was inclined to gain weight. With the *Yogatronic Diet* she controlled her weight, but it was rather flabby and was not adequately protected against turning soft and prematurely middle-aged. To attain your "ideal weight" is but part of the benefit of the *Yogatronic Diet*. The other part consists mainly of doing a certain amount of exercise regularly enough, as advised by the life insurance companies.

Mrs. Young's friends and the media of that time, however, frightened her from exercising vigorously at her age. With her *Yogatronic Diet* and her resulting continuous "ideal weight," I tried to assure her she had little to worry about for she was healthy otherwise. She had been a good swimmer in high school, and she started swimming again. I persuaded her to train and compete in the coming annual *Chicago Tribune* swim meet, particularly in the grueling, super-energy requiring 100-yard dash. The other contestants averaged between 15 and 17 years in age: the age of the majority of Olympic winners and world record holders in swimming. The examining physician at the event was obviously surprised at encountering anyone of Mrs. Young's age even daring to compete in it, and cautiously subjected her to a double examination intermingled with questions of apprehension.

The leading competitors belonged to famous swimming clubs and had trained, on the average, from four to five hours a day. They had been competing in the event for years and even trained in pools to be skillful at turning. Mrs. Young, because of a lack of time, had trained in Lake Michigan only two hours a day for three weeks, because it was still cold late in the spring.

But, she had perfected the *Yogatronic Diet* secret of how to multiply the nutritive value of the devitalized supermarket food she ate, *without adding food supplements*. She felt so strong by the day of the event that she captured the silver medal in her heat against the 16-year old state champion (whose father was a leading coach), who promptly went on to win the event for the second or third year in a row and equalled or broke her own record.

Mrs. Young was still so strong after the exhausting meet that she traveled back to the lake that afternoon and engaged in a full, two-hour strenuous swimming workout. She had proved to herself that she was *even stronger* at 37 than she had been at 16 or 17, thanks mainly to the *Yogatronic Diet*. At my urging she took up jogging regularly, decades before it became a fad. Today, near 70, she still runs outdoors from five to seven miles a day, five days a week.

How Dinah L. Lost Her Big Waist in Record Time, Safely and Naturally

For years, Dinah L. had tried numerous ways to lose her big waist without imperiling her health, but she had given up in despair. With her health still good, she asked me whether the *Yogatronic Diet* could help her, or whether she ought to accept a sizeable waist as a natural part of her. From my nearly 50 years of maintaining the ideal weight (which also includes a normal-sized waist), I replied, "Let your waist lose its shape, and you lose the elegance of your figure, no matter how shapely you may be otherwise. You appear older and lose your flexibility and endurance in sports. You lose sex-appeal and confidence in yourself and no longer feel light and limber. Nor does your health remain at its best. Excess weight around your 'belly' indicates that you are depositing life-shortening fats in your heart, kidneys and arteries."

I told Dinah that, at 40, I had reduced my 33-inch waist to 30 inches in only six weeks without fasts or pills. As she was healthy and not under professional care, the safest way to reduce her waist, I went on, *was* without pills, special diet or surgery, as I myself had done nearly 30 years before. Scientists at the University of Mississippi today support me with similar conclusions. They experimented with a 25-year old restaurant worker, and he lost 219 pounds in just 18 weeks. They affirm that it constitutes a record. The subject lost up to 22 pounds a week, and in 33 weeks, his waist had shrunk from an elephantine 50 inches to a trim 32. Other volunteers followed with similar success.

(*Note*: Not everybody possesses the same build nor the same length of alimentary tract. That explains why no two persons will gain or lose weight at exactly the same pace. Every weight-losing time given here—or in any source, for that matter—must be viewed as a guideline, not as an exact figure to be followed or expected to occur to the letter).

Dinah followed the *Yogatronic Diet* eagerly, and her weight melted off day after day. She lost six inches off her waist in about 13 weeks but reduced her face and the rest of her body "just enough." She took up jogging, but the *Yogatronic Diet* spared her from being cursed with the "stringy, aged jogger's look" in her face and body, which she dreaded.

How Ambrose P. Looked from 15 to 20 Years Younger

Ambrose P. had reached the age at which people accepted him as being no longer young, and he was getting older every year. "I live today, only once," he sighed. "When I was young I had little money. I make good money now, but I have little youth. If I were still young, how different my life would be! Could one but make his youth last forever!"

"We all lose some of it," I agreed with him, "but you can regain a good portion of it. Everybody should make the Fountain of Youth a primary goal in life. To live long and be healthy is to stay younger, for you approach death when you lose too much youth. Maintaining your ideal weight helps to maintain your youth—so long as it is toned-up weight. The wise eating of the *Yogatronic Diet* helps me to maintain both."

I taught Ambrose the *Yogatronic Diet* and the secret of arousing *Power Yoga* assimilation from the outer limits of the skin to the inner cells of his body to reverse the aging process. I taught him how to burst with health, even on supermarket or grocery food, without adding vitamin-minerals, polyunsaturated oils or other food concentrates. I taught him how to neutralize the cumulative effects of the poison chemicals added to his commercial food but remain healthy, vigorous and youthful—even when he drew near 70. I taught him how to raise his alpha-cholesterol, the wonder beneficial cholesterol and how to retain his "ideal" weight. All of this special knowledge is presented in the chapters that follow.

Promptly after commencing the *Yogatronic Diet*, Ambrose noticed the "tremendous change" in his bowel movements. That "change" in itself, he said, made him feel "like a youth" again. In four weeks, his waist "looked lean," yet his face looked fuller. When your bowels move easily and normally, I had long discovered, your face fills up to normalcy. When they move hard and with difficulty, rings form under your eyes and your cheeks are drawn, even though your waistline bulges.

In two weeks, Ambrose's cheeks glowed red with returning youth. The raw beets and the fibrous mass in the *Yogatronic Diet* were already at work and his bowels moved fully and easily. The tension left his face, and the crow's feet at the corners of his eyes were less distinct, bringing back still more the look of youth about him. Invisible changes also took place within his body and showed up in his movements, his walk, his alertness and general demeanor. In two months, Ambrose looked five years younger than he was. In one year he appeared 15 years younger to many strangers.

"*Now* I can make up for the years I missed!" he exclaimed to me, bursting with excitement. I didn't know exactly what he meant by that, but I do know that he had reversed the aging process with the *Yogatronic Diet*.

The Importance of the "Ideal" Weight

Life insurance companies depend much for their success on the accuracy of their screening physicians. Their physicians never fail to compare your weight with that of an ideal composite of healthy persons about your own height, age and type of build. Such a weight is accepted as being the most promising for a long life. It represents the most efficient distribution of your body weight throughout your anatomy. In other words, it is the most advantageous weight for your heart to pump your blood, for your digestive system to feed, for your urinary organs to empty your wastes, for your lungs to supply you with oxygen, for your muscles to move, for your bones to bear, for your nervous system to stimulate, for your mind to find harmony with.

Renowned athletes, like Arnold Schwarzenegger, Muhammad Ali and so many others, add from 30 to 50 pounds to the insurance company's ideal weights for them, in order to compete successfully in their sports. They make every effort to retain this excess weight throughout their careers—or lose their dominance in them. This vastly excess weight is put on with abnormal doses of vitamins and minerals, fantastic muscle-growing anabolic steroids, dangerously concentrated body building foods (like high proteins) or the like. No matter how this excess weight is added, it is still excess weight for the natural heart, digestive organs (including the liver), urinary organs (including the kidneys and bladder), skeletal structure (including the joints, the bones and the spine), for the inherited muscles, for the normal nervous drive.

The Traumas of Added Extraordinary Muscle

Ambitious athletes like these, abnormally subject their bodies and nervous systems to rigors for which they are not naturally capable. They are risking eventual suffering from arthritis from worn down joints, regularly overstrained muscles which could degenerate into muscular dystrophy, liver disease resulting from its detoxification of excess intakes of proteins or other body building foods, kidney and bladder dysfunctions (resulting from ridding the body of excessive wastes), glandular atrophies (caused by prolonged intakes of body building hormones, like anabolic steroids), arthritis of the spine (due to their regularly resisting abnormal powers or weights) and of elbows and knees (resulting from the wearing out of the cartilage caps of these joints) and high blood pressure (brought about by the nervous anxiety of do-or-die competition). For some time, their bodies might not be conscious of ill effects from these traumas, but they may suddenly find themselves crippled for the rest of their lives.

The Disintegration of Being Underweight

The insurance companies are equally wary about the underweight. Researchers have found that your body is not healthiest when you are 10% above, or 10% below, your "ideal" weight, down to the very pound and ounce. My wife, my private disciple and I maintain our ideal weights *all year* round—and do so by "eating like horses" every day. To become extremely underweight like the leading marathon runners, is to lose too much fat from your body.

1. Your joints need fat to maintain their normal lubrication—or you invite arthritis. Too little fat on your face and skin curses you with an early "old age look."
2. Losing too much muscle tissue (which occurs when you are underweight) results in "skinny" arms, legs, back and shoulders and robs you of shape and symmetry.
3. Losing too much fat within your eyeballs causes them to sink into their sockets, to lose their shiny glitter and suggest a corpse's likeness.
4. Your blood pressure may fall too low and leave you prone to fatigue.
5. You feel chilly more easily, and are consequently more nervous and tense. Warmth relaxes, chilliness tenses.
6. Your bones, joints and muscles move about a lighter body mass than they are naturally prepared to and atrophy from "disuse."

The Incomparable Advantages of the "Ideal" Weight

With a permanent "ideal" weight, however, your face and body are covered with the most beautifying amount of fat and muscle possible for their structure and your waist is kept down to the "ideal" size. At your ideal weight you automatically look your best. Principally because of maintaining my "ideal" weight, I am able, at nearly 70 years of age, to continue looking far younger than I am. Old friends who have not seen me, sometimes for as long as 30 years, invariably remark when they meet me again, "I can't believe it! You haven't aged a day!" The well known columnist, Jeff

Lyon, interviewed me a year ago for the "Close Up" column in the *Chicago Tribune* and wrote, "Some say Dr. Young is 66 years old. He looks far younger." I look far younger at my "ideal" weight because at such a weight my body mass is distributed most evenly all over, both in function and looks. At such a weight, your whole body will operate most efficiently, like a well-oiled, safely cargo-loaded machine. No part of it will be naturally *overused* or *under-burdened.* No part of it will suffer unnecessarily at the expense of another and suffer from a premature malfunction.

Your "ideal" weight is also the best and easiest weight for you to maintain day-after-day with the *Yogatronic Diet*—and yet you "eat like a horse." With it, you don't have to become "grossly overweight" when you don't exercise over a long period of time, as Muhammad Ali apparently does. At different periods of my life, I have hardly exercised for as long as a year. But I did *not gain a pound*, nor did I lose my best physical size. With the *Yogatronic Diet*, neither will you. Yet, Arnold Swartzenegger admits that since retiring from body building he has lost 20 pounds or more, and that he has not had his body measured for years because, obviously, he no longer possesses his once spectacular measurements. But, on my diet, although I never fatten or shrink, even when I take extensive layoffs, although I lose in muscle tone, of course, I regain it when I resume exercise and swiftly look my best again. All during the long lay off, however, my face and body retain their "ideal" weight symmetry and keep me looking my handsomest and youngest.

These secrets will be revealed in this book, the *Yogatronic Diet*.

THE "IDEAL" WEIGHT—THE PROVED SECRET OF LONG LIFE, ENDURING HEALTH, AND LASTING BEAUTY

The Nearly 40 Year Researched and Proved Table of "Ideal Weights"

On page 28 are the latest tables issued by the Metropolitan Life Insurance Company, revealing the "IDEAL" weights (also called "DESIRABLE" weights), for you to seek, according to your height and frame.

DESIRABLE WEIGHTS FOR MEN AND WOMEN
According to Height and Frame, Ages 25 and Over

HEIGHT (in Shoes)*	SMALL FRAME	MEDIUM FRAME	LARGE FRAME
	Weight in Pounds (In Indoor Clothing)		
MEN			
5' 2"	112-120	118-129	126-141
3"	115-123	121-133	129-144
4"	118-126	124-136	132-148
5"	121-129	127-139	135-152
6"	124-133	130-143	138-156
7"	128-137	134-147	142-161
8"	132-141	138-152	147-166
9"	136-145	142-156	151-170
10"	140-150	146-160	155-174
11"	144-154	150-165	159-179
6' 0"	148-158	154-170	164-184
1"	152-162	158-175	168-189
2"	156-167	162-180	173-194
3"	160-171	167-185	178-199
4"	164-175	172-190	182-204
WOMEN			
4' 10"	92- 98	96-107	104-119
11"	94-101	98-110	106-122
5' 0"	96-104	101-113	109-125
1"	99-107	104-116	112-128
2"	102-110	107-119	115-131
3"	105-113	110-122	118-134
4"	108-116	113-126	121-138
5"	111-119	116-130	125-142
6"	114-123	120-135	129-146
7"	118-127	124-139	133-150
8"	122-131	128-143	137-154
9"	126-135	132-147	141-158
10"	130-140	136-151	145-163
11"	134-144	140-155	149-168
6' 0"	138-148	144-159	153-173

*1-inch heels for men and 2-inch heels for women.

Note: Prepared by the Metropolitan Life Insurance Company. Derived primarily from data of the *Build and Blood Pressure Study, 1959*, Society of Actuaries.

How the Latest Findings of the 110-Year Researchers of Nearly 10,000,000 People Continue to Substantiate Yogatronics

As this book goes to press, the Association of Life Insurance Medical Directors and the Society of Actuaries issued their latest 20-year Build and Blood Pressure Study. It is the sequel to the one issued 20 years ago, from which the Metropolitan Life Insurance Company developed the Ideal Weight chart on the preceding page, which you are to use as your weight guide. These two studies cover a total of 44 years of insurance company experience. The table of the new Study is reproduced on the next two pages with the special permissions of the researchers. Actuaries produce these tables and life insurance companies use them to determine which applicants are insurable. These tables are the basis of the desirable ("ideal") weight tables used by the life insurance companies and doctors, and are printed on coin-operated scales. Edward A. Lew, the actuary who directed the latest study, as well as the previous one so many years ago when he was with the Metropolitan Life Insurance Company, states that "high blood pressure and overweight" either alone or together, remain "significant causes of excess mortality" among insured populations. These studies were actually initiated in 1869, combining 10,000,000 people.

The new weight table investigated more than 4,000,000 persons. It discovered that the average young person of today is heavier than such a person was 25 years ago, because of "better nutrition." But Mr. Lew explained that the "average" weights are *not* the same as "desirable" (or "Ideal") weights. "Ideal" weight, he said, would be about 7% *below* the "average" weight, and synchronizes with the "lowest death rate" for a specific height. This wealth of 44 years of statistics was derived from millions and millions of people and coincides with the ideal weight results of the Yogatronic Diet. And yet, I published the condensed version of this diet four full years before the results of the *first* study of this 110-year incontrovertible record was published.

Important: In the table of the new study, notice that the average weights at 50-59 years are between 16 and 24 lbs. heavier than those at 20-24. Yet, with the Yogatronic Diet I easily keep my weight exactly what it was at my ideal weight at 20, and yet eat like a horse and never fast.

1979 BUILD & BLOOD PRESSURE STUDY

Average weights of men
Graduated weight in shoes and indoor clothing in pounds

	15-16 years			17-19 years			20-24 years			25-29 years			30-39 years			40-49 years			50-59 years			60-69 years		
Height	1959 study	1979 study	Weight change	1959 study	1979 study	Weight change	1959 study	1979 study	Weight change	1959 study	1979 study	Weight change	1959 study	1979 study	Weight change	1959 study	1979 study	Weight change	1959 study	1979 study	Weight change	1959 study	1979 study	Weight change
5′ 2″	107	112	+ 5	119	128	+ 9	128	137	+ 9	134	140	+ 6	137	142	+ 5	140	142	+ 2	142	141	− 1	139	140	+ 1
3″	112	116	+ 5	123	129	+ 6	132	136	+ 4	138	141	+ 3	141	143	+ 2	144	144	0	145	145	0	142	144	+ 2
4″	117	121	+ 4	127	132	+ 5	136	139	+ 3	141	143	+ 2	145	147	+ 2	148	149	+ 1	149	150	+ 1	146	149	+ 3
5″	122	127	+ 5	131	137	+ 6	139	143	+ 4	144	147	+ 3	149	151	+ 2	152	154	+ 2	153	155	+ 2	150	153	+ 3
6″	127	133	+ 6	135	141	+ 6	142	148	+ 6	148	152	+ 4	153	156	+ 3	156	158	+ 2	157	159	+ 2	154	158	+ 4
7″	132	137	+ 5	139	145	+ 6	145	153	+ 8	151	156	+ 5	157	160	+ 3	161	163	+ 2	162	164	+ 2	159	163	+ 4
8″	137	143	+ 6	143	150	+ 7	149	157	+ 8	155	161	+ 6	161	164	+ 4	165	167	+ 2	166	168	+ 2	163	167	+ 4
9″	142	148	+ 6	147	155	+ 8	153	162	+10	159	166	+ 7	165	170	+ 5	169	172	+ 3	170	173	+ 3	168	172	+ 4
10″	146	153	+ 7	151	159	+ 8	157	167	+10	163	171	+ 8	170	174	+ 4	174	176	+ 2	175	177	+ 2	173	176	+ 3
11″	150	159	+ 9	155	164	+ 9	161	171	+10	167	175	+ 8	174	179	+ 5	178	181	+ 3	180	182	+ 2	178	181	+ 3
6′ 0″	154	162	+ 8	160	168	+ 8	166	176	+10	172	181	+ 9	179	184	+ 5	183	186	+ 3	185	187	+ 2	183	186	+ 3
1″	159	168	+ 9	164	174	+10	170	182	+12	177	186	+ 9	183	190	+ 7	187	192	+ 5	189	183	+ 4	188	191	+ 3
2″	164	173	+ 9	168	179	+ 9	174	187	+13	182	191	+ 9	188	195	+ 7	192	197	+ 5	194	198	+ 4	193	196	+ 3
3″	169	178	+ 9	172	185	+13	178	193	+15	186	197	+11	193	201	+ 8	197	203	+ 6	199	204	+ 5	198	200	+ 2
4″	175	184	+ 9	176	190	+14	181	198	+17	190	202	+12	199	206	+ 7	203	208	+ 5	205	209	+ 4	204	207	+ 3

Average weights of women
Graduated weight in shoes and indoor clothing in pounds

	15-16 years			17-19 years			20-24 years			25-29 years			30-39 years			40-49 years			50-59 years			60-69 years		
Height	1959 study	1979 study	Weight change	1959 study	1979 study	Weight change	1959 study	1979 study	Weight change	1959 study	1979 study	Weight change	1959 study	1979 study	Weight change	1959 study	1979 study	Weight change	1959 study	1979 study	Weight change	1959 study	1979 study	Weight change
4′ 10″	97	101	+ 4	99	103	+ 4	102	105	− 3	107	110	+ 3	115	113	− 2	122	118	− 4	125	121	− 4	127	123	− 4
11″	100	105	+ 5	102	108	+ 6	105	110	+ 5	110	112	+ 2	117	115	− 2	124	121	− 3	127	125	− 2	129	127	− 2
5′ 0″	103	109	+ 6	105	111	+ 6	108	112	+ 4	113	114	+ 1	120	118	− 2	127	123	− 4	130	127	− 3	131	130	− 1
1″	107	112	+ 5	109	115	+ 6	112	116	+ 4	116	119	+ 3	123	121	− 2	130	127	− 3	133	131	− 2	134	133	− 1
2″	111	117	+ 6	113	119	+ 6	115	120	+ 5	119	121	+ 2	126	124	− 2	133	129	− 4	136	133	− 3	137	136	− 1
3″	114	121	+ 7	116	123	+ 7	118	124	+ 6	122	125	+ 3	129	128	− 1	136	133	− 3	140	137	− 3	141	140	− 1
4″	117	123	+ 6	120	126	+ 6	121	127	+ 6	125	128	+ 3	132	131	− 1	140	136	− 4	144	141	− 3	145	143	− 2
5″	121	128	+ 7	124	129	+ 5	125	130	+ 5	129	132	+ 3	135	134	− 1	143	139	− 4	148	144	− 4	149	147	− 2
6″	125	131	+ 6	127	132	+ 5	129	133	+ 4	133	134	+ 1	139	137	− 2	147	143	− 4	152	147	− 5	153	150	− 3
7″	128	135	+ 7	130	136	+ 6	132	137	+ 5	136	138	+ 2	142	141	− 1	151	147	− 4	156	152	− 4	157	155	− 2
8″	132	138	+ 6	134	140	+ 6	136	141	+ 5	140	142	+ 2	146	145	− 1	155	150	− 5	160	156	− 4	161	158	− 3
9″	136	142	+ 6	138	145	+ 7	140	146	+ 6	144	148	+ 4	150	150	0	159	155	− 4	164	159	− 5	165	161	− 4
10″	*	146	—	142	148	+ 6	144	149	+ 5	148	150	+ 2	154	153	− 1	164	158	− 6	169	162	− 7	*	163	—
11″	*	149	—	147	150	+ 3	149	155	+ 6	153	156	+ 3	159	159	0	169	162	− 7	174	166	− 8	*	167	—
6 0″	*	152	—	152	154	+ 2	154	157	+ 3	158	159	+ 1	164	164	0	174	168	− 6	180	171	− 9	*	172	—

The 1959 Build and Blood Pressure Study reflects data collected during the years 1935 through 1954. The 1979 Build and Blood Pressure Study reflects data collected during the years from 1954 through 1972

SOURCE: Ad Hoc Committee of the New Build and Blood Pressure Study Association of America and Society of Actuaries

Here is the simple way to pinpoint your "ideal" weight from the table "Ideal Weight," page 28.

1. If you are a man, look for your barefoot height and build on it. Then *subtract* about two pounds from the range of given weights.
2. If you are a woman, find your barefoot height and build on it. *Add* 1 inch to that height. Look at the weight given for it and *add* about 1-1/2 pounds.

Don't cheat or fool yourself in the computation. Your life, health and personal handsomeness (or beauty) is at stake. The weights in the "ideal" tables issued by the Metropolitan Life Insurance Company over the last 36 years vary only three pounds or less from one another. Other tables will be issued from time to time, but the difference in the weights will obviously be negligible. So, you can confidently rely upon the accuracy of the present one.

Study your own weight in it now. Then follow the *Yogatronic Diet*, eat "like a horse" and look and feel young all your life, even when near 70. I spent a whole lifetime experimenting on myself to find the secret of long life, health and youth preservation and have reaped the benefits in a trim youthful build. I promise you similar results from *Yogatronics*.

The Nucleus of the Secret

Your waistline is the secret axis of your every achievement, whether it is physical, mental, psychic, material, romantic, career-oriented, youth-maintaining or health-creating. It is the secret axis for your living an extraordinarily long and healthy life, for your bursting daily with energy, for your being physically powerful or full of endurance, for your personal attractiveness, indeed, for any goal you seek. Let your waist lose its shape and you lose the elegance of your figure, no matter how remarkably you may be developed or how eye-catchingly you are molded otherwise. Instantly, you look older than you are. You lose your flexibility and your endurance in sports. You lose sex appeal. You lose confidence in yourself. You no longer feel light and limber.

Your health does not remain at its best either. Excess weight around your midsection indicates that you are depositing life-shortening fat in your heart, liver, kidneys and arteries.

At 40, with the *Yogatronic Diet*, I reduced my 33 inch waist to 30 in *only six weeks* of steady workouts without weights, fasts, pills or any apparatus. It helped me to place as a finalist in a statewide body-building contest with a youth half my age (22) who had been weight-lifting for years and who held a closetful of trophies in weight lifting and body building. He was in such stupendous shape for the contest that he went on to win the titles of Mr. America, Mr. USA, Mr. World, and Mr. Universe. There are no higher amateur titles to win, and he refused to turn professional. He even swept off all the subdivision trophies like: Best Arms, Best Chest, Best Back, Best Legs, and Most Muscular. He accumulated the highest number of points for his wins since John Grimek.

He accomplished this spectacular record, to repeat, with the help of gulping massive doses of vitamins and body-building pills every day for months. In contrast, I continued with my daily, everyday supermarket food and health-store seaweed because then, as well as now, I refused to subject my body to what I considered the possible risks of concentrated foods.

Your Secret Lever

Your waist, to repeat, is the secret axis, the secret lever to all your achievements, whether within you or outside of you. It contains your solar plexus, the great crossway of your instinctive nervous system (your sympathetics and parasympathetics) which automatically controls your vital functions. Your waist and solar plexus control your breathing, heartbeat, liver and kidneys. They control the digestion, absorption and assimilation of your food; your circulation, body temperature and acid and alkaline balance; your blood pressure and glands; your special senses (that is, your sight, hearing, smell, taste, touch, heat and cold, and your sense of pressure); your sexuality, emotions and the whole gamut of physical senses and functions. Your waist houses either major portions or the whole of most of your visceral organs. It contains the thickest portion of your spinal column, including its most vulnerable joints, like the lumbosacral joint at the base of your spine. Your sciatic nerve originates in your waist and passes downwards.

Your waist (or abdomen) extends down from your rib-box to your hips. It is the seat of most internal growths, hernias and ruptures, and it hosts your appendix and your adrenal glands (your important glands of self-preservation, or of "fight or flight"). Your alimentary tract, which coils all through your waist, receives the fuel food that provides your body with life and transforms it into a physical and chemical form which your body can absorb easiest, assimilate fastest and utilize for energy, repair and growth, or to resist or combat disease and stall ever-threatening death.

Your Waist—Beyond its Function as an Axis

A slim waist, however, does not simply constitute small measurement around the middle. A healthy, small-enough waist proves that you have a vigorous, well-functioning and attractive-looking body. With such a body, your mind can function at its best and release your hidden powers. It prepares you to make miracle discoveries in any field, even without a laboratory, as I have done repeatedly since the age of 10.

When you lose weight mainly from your arms, legs, torso and back, you don't feel as if you are walking on air. But you *do* feel as if you are walking on air when your waist is lean. Your heart, liver, kidneys, stomach and other visceral organs have more space to function, and receive more blood from their less compressed arteries. You hold your rib-box higher, for it is pinioned down by less of a load. Your diaphragm and lungs regain some lost breathing space. Your bowels are emptier, because you can't be eating your fill and still have a slim waist if you are constipated. Your autointoxication dissipates and less blood congests in your splanchnic pool (the mass of veins in your abdomen) leaving more blood available for your muscles and brain.

Your waistline, to put it tersely, is your lifeline. When small and healthy, it is not bloated with gas, except for the temporary gas resulting from the bowel-moving roughage of fibrous foods. Its muscles (for the abdomen is covered with muscles, even if they are concealed by some normal fat) hold your visceral organs in place instead of letting them collapse forwards and downwards upon your pelvis, pushing out your waist and flattening your lower back abnormally (See Illus. 1). Such a kyphotic back curve (even if too slight to be recognized by the untrained eye) pinches the spinal nerves that branch out from your spinal cord, including your pair of

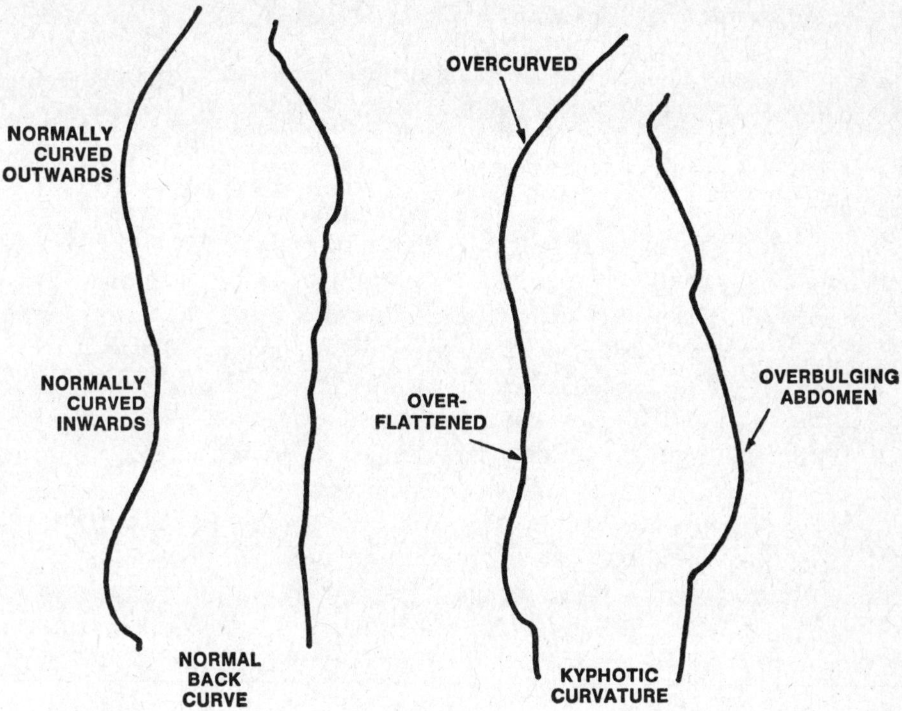

Illustration 1

sciatic nerves. It also constricts blood vessels of your abdomen and pelvis, which convey the blood from your legs back to your lungs and heart. Such a lower-back flattening and abnormal upper-back forward-curving brings you discomfort, detracts from your appearance, plagues you with a feeling of lassitude, pessimism and easy fatigue and can curse you with intermittent constipation and autointoxication.

Such a back-flattening causes your rib-box to drop and squash your stomach. Man or woman, you feel pregnant, but you are pregnant only with congested viscera, with distending gas, with slow-moving putrefying fecal matter. You have less blood being synthesized in your compacted spleen, impaired detoxication of your body impurities in your crushed liver and delayed excretion of your urinary wastes from your strangled kidneys. Your very heart is dislocated slightly to the left and cannot beat at its best, bringing you an "aging look."

The Hazards of Seeking a Small Waist

It is no simple matter to acquire a small waist. Fasting, fad diets and weight-reducing gimmicks can lead to serious disturbances, according to Dr. Dean Fletcher, associate director of the AMA's Department of Food and Nutrition. Among the fad diets are: (1) low-protein diet, (2) high-protein diet, (3) grapefruit diet, (4) diuretic diet (water pills), (5) thyroid hormones, (6) HCG hormones, (7) amphetamines (pep pills), (8) hard-boiled egg diet, (9) liquid formula diets, and a host of others.

The safest fastest way, unless you are not healthy and are under your professional healer's orders, is without pills, special diet or surgery. Science discovered such a way at the University of Mississippi, and it was described at length in the Feb. 2, 1977, *National Enquirer*. By following it, a 25-year old restaurant worker lost 219 pounds in just 38 weeks, which seemed to constitute a record. Dr. Phillip Cooker of the University's educational psychology department made an exhaustive study of behavioral literature and found that it *was* a record. This volunteer and the others who participated in the program were not told what to eat. They had already been given "hundreds" of diets and had not followed them. They were simply told to eat less than they usually ate. Mainly, they were made aware of what they ate, when they ate, how rapidly they ate and how much they ate.

But, they were to eat all their meals at regular times in a particular place. They were to chew and swallow every mouthful carefully before they took another. They were not to read, look at television or listen to music while at the table. Snacks were absolutely forbidden between meals.

The restaurant worker lost up to 22 pounds a week. In 38 weeks his waist had shrunk from an elephantine 50 inches to a trim 32. Once he shed his old eating habits and acquired the new ones, he confessed that it was no problem to continue with them. You can do the same.

Solar Diet—the Record that Broke the Record 23 Years Before Science

The diet the restaurant worker followed is precisely the weight-reducing, waist-trimming "wise eating" program that I had revealed to my readers in the limited edition of my book, *Solar Diet, 23 years earlier.* No wonder the results were unusual and fantastic. In an updating of *Solar Diet's* "wise eating" program, with its thorough explanation of each step, which the science report did not give, I have created the *Yogatronic Diet.*

For the average person, *Yogatronics* does not recommend dieting. It recommends "wise eating." But, neither a correct diet nor wise eating—alone—can be guaranteed to keep you in good health. *How* you eat, what you think of as you eat, what you do *before* and *after* you eat are just as important as *what* you eat.

Yogatronics advises three meals a day, which should be consumed at the same time every day—except on special occasions that make it impossible to do so. By eating regularly you fill your stomach at regular times and induce digestive and peristaltic action at regular times. Eating with regularity is an important contributor to lifelong health and eternal youth.

Regularity also trains your digestive system to anxiously expect to be fed at a certain hour. Precisely at that hour, the glands start secreting slightly, even if no food is put in your stomach. If you eat right then, you catch your stomach at its *digestive prime.*

Furthermore, your tissues, at a precise time after this, are best ready to absorb the right amount of food which your body needs. At that time they won't be overfed or starved, and you are less likely to overeat or undereat.

The Word "Diet" Is Misleading

The word "diet," indeed, is misleading. Diet suggests the starving and limiting of your natural appetite. I consume hearty meals every day, but they are wise meals.

Curbing your appetite, especially by swallowing artificial substances which lessen appetite, fools your taste glands so that they lose much of their ability to let you know what particular foods your system needs most. As a result, you lose weight—but perhaps you also lose your health.

Mealtime regularity spins *rhythm regularity* (which science discovered 15 years after my *Solar Diet* and called bio-rhythm) in your whole system. It is a regularity of prime importance in bringing you a long-lasting life, saturated with the joys of good health. The *Yogatronic Diet* won't convert you into an anxiety-driven health fiend, but it will automatically cast off the degenerative habits in your present way of life which have ruined, or will ruin, your health. *Yogatronics* will transform you with its amazing health secrets, which have turned out to be the *safest natural way to reduce*, according to science's own discovery.

Keep away from all snacks, between meals or before going to bed. Indeed, keep away from all snacks altogether. When you eat, eat well. In between your three meals a day, *don't eat.*

Adding too much taste to any food tends to flood your mouth with saliva and your stomach with digestive juice—all of which can lead to acidosis. The more normal you keep the taste of food, the better it is for your digestion. Your stomach then secretes the *right amount* of juice to digest the food and not an exorbitant amount in response to the artificially created exaggerated taste of the food.

Now you know *what* to eat, *when* to eat, *what not* to eat and *when not* to eat. Learn, next, *how* to eat your food.

What to do With Your Mind When You Eat

A belief also existed that you had to chew your food slowly. Fast chewing was said to cause indigestion. Yogatronics considers that belief hocum. Your chewing speed has nothing to do with your food digestion. As long as your food is broken down to fine bits and mixed thoroughly with your saliva before it is swallowed, that is sufficient. Whether this is accomplished faster or slower in the mouth makes little difference as far as digestion is concerned. As far as your saliva mixing with your food is concerned, it mixes just as fast with it whether you chew slowly or quickly. Saliva, after all, is practically a liquid. What the anti-fast-chewing faddists really meant was, "Chew your food for a *long time.* Don't bolt it down!" But the public misinterpreted the ambiguous use of the word "slow" in the warning and started *chewing* slowly, and long, drawn-out chewing ruined the pleasure of eating. Everybody won't chew at the same speed, no more than everybody will talk or run at the same speed. Eat at your own natural pace . . .

But there *is* some harm in conversing during most of the meal and hardly thinking about the meal itself, hardly tasting anything but the first mouthful. Those who speak too much while they eat, end up eating very little. It is not because they have no appetite, but because their attention divides itself between the food and the conversation.

If you are trying to reduce, this might seem like the solution to your problem, but it is not. To reduce, you have to *change* the kind of food you eat, to stop eating food that turns to fat. But you still have to eat good meals; you still have to put bulky, healthy food into your system, or you starve yourself and become constipated.

Eating Wisely Is A Tremendous Achievement

Eating is a big project in itself. Like other natural performances, to do it best you have to do it with your attention focused completely on it. When you eat, eating is the important thing. To deprive it of your full attention, will result in your performing it half-heartedly. Attention cannot be divided; it can only be alternated from one activity to another. It is believed by many that you ought to be happy when you eat, and that you ought to laugh and enjoy yourself. That belief is true in regards to your frame of mind when you eat. But *keep your attention* primarily *on your food.* When eating, avoid discussions which completely absorb your mind or even similarly gripping jokes. Light, even romantic, banter draws your attention less from your food than serious conversation. A group at the table adds pleasantly to the serious conversation, but the meal should remain the most important consideration.

Don't let long discussions prolong dinner time endlessly. Also, the cook should not take so long to serve the different dishes that the stomachs of the diners digest the early dishes thoroughly before the later dishes. Both situations ruin the appetites of the diners. The dishes should be served and eaten steadily, one after another, for best results. *Then* everybody can sit back in their chairs and talk their heads off in pleasant conversation, discussion or fun, but not in heated argument. During and after the meal, use the utmost diplomacy to make it a thrilling experience, divorcing it from the stark issues of the day.

The information on "wise eating" which you have just read is the part of *Yogatronics* based on my original Solar Diet. You can see how *exactly*, step-by-step, the program of *Solar Diet* was like the record-breaking weight-losing diet discovery at the University of Mississippi described to the world *twenty-three years later*, in which the 25-year old restaurant worker lost a record 219 pounds in 38 weeks, without pills, special diet or surgery! Not only did I *discover* this program 40 years before, and *publish* it 23 years before science proved it, but I did so without a laboratory.

The Secret Beyond the Record-Breaking Weight-Reducing Program

In *Solar Diet* I had already gone *beyond* the record-breaking weight-losing discovery made at the University. In it, I described in detail every step from getting up in the morning to going to bed, a total of about 20,000 words. Science has announced only the general conclusions it has formed after examining the results of its experiment. It will take many more long experiments for it to work out the exact details. So, *Solar Diet*, although published 23 years ahead of science, is still farther ahead of the time. Yet, up to now, you have barely tapped the ocean of wise-eating secrets which will be revealed to you in the *Yogatronics* diet.

"The Power of Suggestion in Eating"

Everything you eat does you more good when you *believe in the food* and imagine that it does for you exactly what it is supposed to do. The pessimist injures only himself and those who believe in his jibes. When you swallow your glass of warm water and lemon juice in the morning, visualize it flowing down your esophagus into your stomach and neutralizing its contents. Then visualize it flowing on into your intestine, through its walls into your bloodstream and into your liver and kidneys. Visualize it purifying your blood and cleaning your tissues. Visualize it neutralizing the acid in your stomach and bringing you an appetite for a big, hearty breakfast.

The Best Way to Eat

When eating, try to put every thought out of your mind, except that of the taste and delight of the food before you. Absorb yourself completely in every mouthful of it. Even after you swallow it, momentarily visualize all the good it is doing your body. If you have just swallowed fruits and vegetables, visualize them alkalizing your blood and refueling your system with vitality. If you have just swallowed meat, visualize it building up your muscles. The power of the mind goes a long way to encourage everything you eat to do exactly what you hope it will do. Let your mind aid your digestion at every step. Let it help direct the food you eat to do its duty more easily. Do your duty to yourself, and try to eat with all-absorbed relish, not with divided attention. The best food in the world will not do miracles for you, unless your mind helps. When your mind helps, only God knows what miracles you can accomplish.

How much faster might the 25-year old restaurant worker of the record breaking weight-reducing program conducted at the University of Mississippi have lost weight had he added this last step of *Yogatronics* to his behavior modification program! As it was, he lost weight with the physical and mental alone, not with the psychic in addition. So, science has not yet caught up with the whole of *Yogatronics'* reducing secrets. But you will do so *right now*, starting with the next chapter.

2

the triple tonic secret

How to Extract More Nutrition from Your Food Through Odic Force

In the 24 years following the publishing of *Solar Diet* I have leaped another 24 years ahead of present-day science. With the *Yogatronic Diet*, I have expanded *Solar Diet* to six times its length and have added to it the miracle-making Triple Tonic Secret.

By masticating and visualizing your food, as you just read at the end of the last chapter, you absorb more completely the odic force of each particular food. The *odic force* is an emanation present in every substance, living or dead. (Illus. 2). It was discovered by Baron von Reichenbach in 1848 and is developed for psychic healing in my recent book, *Zodic Force Control: Secret of Miracle Healing and Long Life.*[1] You extract the utmost nutrition out of every food you eat, through its odic force.

The odic force of the food is transferred to your body through contact, as Reichenbach discovered. But the transfer, which is a characteristic of odic force, does not occur swiftly. It requires up to several minutes to complete. You can't wait that long to chew each mouthful of food, so you better shred or grate most of your food before you eat it. You thereby expose far more surface of the food to saliva in your mouth and to your hydrochloric acid and enzymes

THE ODIC FORCE

ANY
SUBSTANCE
LIVING
OR
DEAD
EMANATES
AN INVISIBLE
ODIC FORCE.
IT IS NOT
THE AURA,
FOR IT REMAINS
WITH THE
SUBSTANCES
ALWAYS.
BUT IT CHANGES WITH
TEMPERATURE AND OTHER
INFLUENCES.

Illustration 2

in your stomach and intestines. Your food, as a result, transfers more of its odic force to your body. That is the *physical* method to extract more odic force from your food.

The Discovery of the Russian Scientists to Double the Length of Your Life

Lastly, subject your food to the Triple Tonic Secret and *double its effectiveness* on your body. In my long interview with Jeff Lyon for his "Close Up" column in the *Chicago Tribune* Sunday edition[2], I announced that I expected to live to 330 years old or longer. Nearly a million readers considered that ridiculous. A week later, however, the *Los Angeles Times* reported that Russian scientists believed that human beings could not only live 100 years, but up to *400 years or longer*.[3] The Russians had experimentally doubled the life span of houseflies by feeding them *magnetized sugar*. A magnet forces all the molecules in the substance it magnetizes to point in the same direction. (See Illus. 3B) like soldiers in a column.

That experiment followed the lines of thought presented in the Triple Tonic Secret. I had originated the idea in *Solar Diet* by explaining (as you read in the last chapter) how to visualize your food as you ate it. Two hundred years ago, leading scientists had

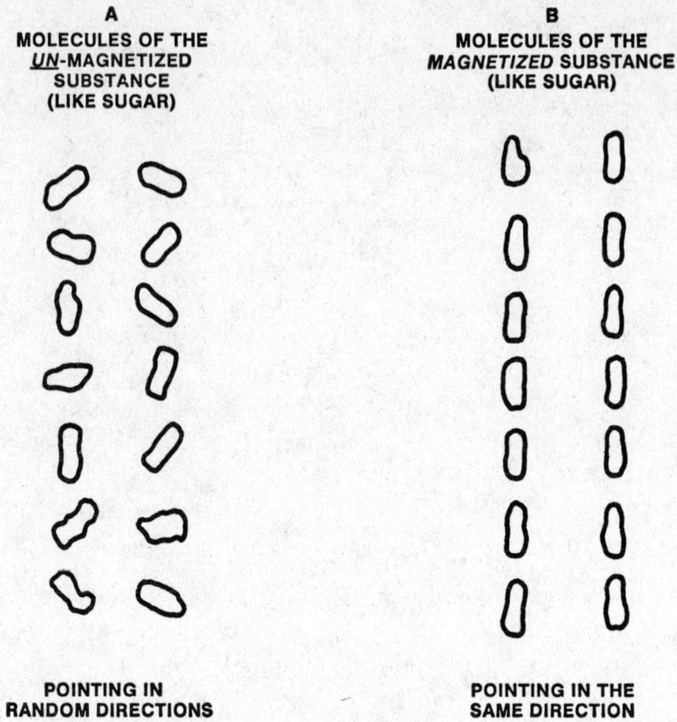

Illustration 3

run Mesmer out of Paris for healing with magnetism, but in 1977 respected Russian scientists were doubling the life span of houseflies with *magnetized sugar*! (See Illus. 3). I, however, had revealed in *Solar Diet*, 23 years before the Russians, how to substantially increase the power of the mind to "magnetize" food and have developed that power far more with the Triple Tonic Secret as fully described in the *Yogatronic Diet*. You will learn that secret now.

The Urgent Need for the Triple Tonic Secret

Despite my spending a lifetime studying foods and diets, as well as inheriting almost 200 years worth of food knowledge from my Yogi and medical and dental ancestors, I was panic-stricken by the mass of dangerous alterations which modern civilization and commercialism were effecting on food and their dire threats to one's very health and life. From my seventeenth year on, I had lived continuously in heavily polluted metropolises, like New

York, Chicago and Los Angeles, except for two brief stays of about five months each in small towns. Living mostly in old apartment buildings, not too far from the crowded downtown areas, there was no practical way for me to grow my own food anywhere.

I subsisted, instead, on the food sold in big city grocery stores and supermarkets. They offered food that was grown on depleted soil, flooded with natural and synthetic dyes, processed, degenerated, frozen, stored much too long and saturated with layers of pesticides. It had lost an alarming percentage of its vitamin content. It was picked green and forced to ripen with gas, and was fumigated and bleached. This food had the vitamin-packed germ removed and had been subjected to emulsifiers and solidifiers, homogenized, artificially colored and flavored, treated with nitric acid with sometimes as much as 400% more preservative chemicals added. It had been robbed of minerals, de-branned and polished. That was just the beginning; processed food was also saturated with autooxidants of fats, lipoids and vegetable matters, sweeteners, surfactants (detergents, foaming agents), water conditioners (iodine, fluoride), humectants (smoke agents), chemical sterilizing agents, antifoaming agents, salt substitutes, shortening, softeners, modifiers and improvers (meat tenderizers and the like), oil and fat substitutes, organic solvents, pesticide residues, insect repellents, hormonal fattening agents, anti-sprouting agents of fruits and vegetables, antibiotics (fed to animals and added to foods), chemical sterilizing agents, wrapping and coating materials (paraffins, waxes, resins, plastics), enzymes, antienzymes, silicones, mineral oils, pollutants, soot glued to smoked foodstuffs and "roasted and toasted" nutriments, household detergents and their coloring chemicals and radiation and radioactive products assimilated by plants and food animals from air, soil or water contaminated by radioactive fall-out. New chemicals and other processes were being added regularly to the seemingly endless parade of "food killers." How could I, or anyone else, expect to be healthy and survive to a vigorous old age while being flushed daily with such death-dealing concoctions?

The food companies' answer was that fresh foods spoil too fast, and they cannot be rushed to the consumer fast enough. The nation, they said, can be fed only with technology—or with processed foods.

Their answer could not be disputed. Still, I had to eat to stay alive! To subsist solely on organically grown foods was outside my modest means. The inflated prices of the grocery and supermarket food counters were impoverishing me enough! Even then, the farmer claimed that he was working for nothing and demanded more profit. How could I save myself and my wife from inevitable disaster? How could billions of other people save themselves from the same fate? The solution was the Triple Tonic Secret.

The Secret Detonator of the Triple Tonic Secret

The use of mind power I had described in *Solar Diet* gave me the clue. With it, I would *multiply* the values of the lost nutrients of the foods I ate. Simultaneously, I would nullify the effects of the toxins that had been added to them. The result would be a decisive increase in the magnetization of the beneficial aspects of the food (as Mesmer achieved with the sick part when he used the magnet to treat disease). I would use the odic force as the magnet.

When foods were mistreated, as they were by chemicals and other means, and lost much of their nutrient value, their uniformly pointing molecules were thrown into disarray, like those of cancer cells. (Illus. 3A). Mesmer's magnets healed, apparently, by realigning the molecules of sick tissues. But it would be easier, I concluded, to normalize the distorted odic forces of my mistreated foods and implant their normalized odic forces into the psychic cells of my tissues. That would revitalize my physical body and endow it with a semblance of immortality. My body would become immune to the deadly effects of the unavoidable food poisons!

The Lobe of Psychic Wisdom

After several years of further study of anatomy and the nervous system in professional graduate school for my doctorate, I traced the detonation point for such a fantastic power. It turned out to be the intermediate lobe of the pituitary gland. (Illus. 4). I had discovered "the lobe of psychic wisdom." Although it is rudimentary in man, it increases with size and age (Rasmussen).[4] Being almost bloodless, according to Gray's *Anatomy*, it is not fed by the body. In man it is supposed to have no function, but *lives by itself* and is subject to little or no living force. I realized, however, that it was *subject to a psychic force.*

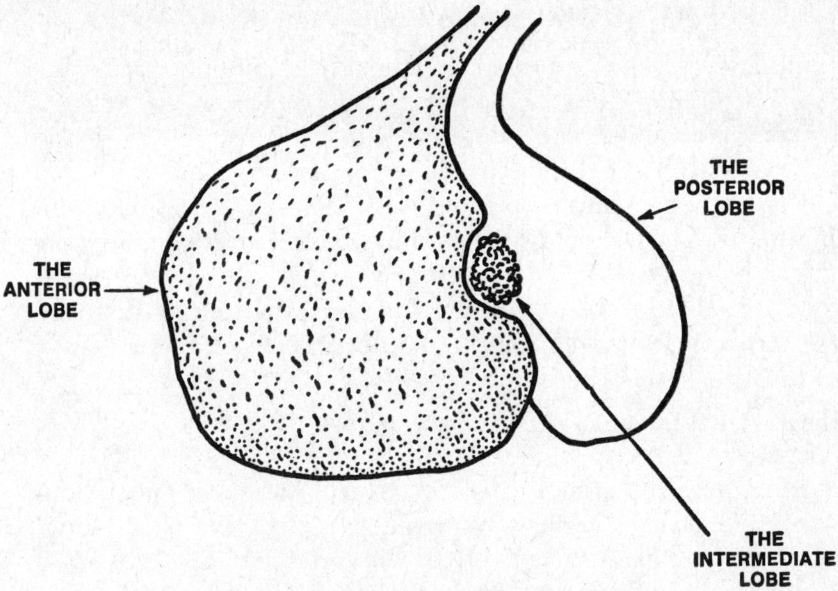

THE 3 LOBES OF YOUR PITUITARY GLAND

Illustration 4

Since the size of the intermediate lobe of the pituitary increased with age, in order to make it perform the miracle of approaching immortality you would have to keep it as small and as much supplied with blood as possible. You could do so only by *using* it through physical and psychic means—or both. It is separate from the anterior lobe and seems to be more of a part of the posterior lobe than of the anterior. (See Illus. 4).

In man, it remains as a thin sheet of skin, with (to repeat) little or no blood supply. Although its function was unknown, some investigators claimed that it had a *stimulating action on the intestinal muscle*.

That was a historic clue! As the intermediate lobe appeared to be more a part of the posterior lobe of the pituitary than of the anterior, I studied the posterior lobe. This lobe contains an extract, pituitrin, which constricts blood vessels. It also brings about a general contraction of smooth (instinctive) muscle throughout the body, which includes the muscle of the *intestines*. Stimulating the intermediate lobe strongly enough, then, would intensify the contraction of my intestines during digestion!

How Your Intermediate Lobe Ages You Prematurely

The cells of the intermediate lobe of your pituitary gland provide the (driving force) of the posterior lobe of the gland.[5] When you advance in years, the intermediate lobe casts off more and more of its cells, and they invade the posterior lobe of the gland and are changed into "senile cells."[6] They doom you and your pituitary to an earlier old age by robbing your intestinal muscles of tone. These muscles contract less firmly then and allow your digesting food to form hard masses. Even if not obvious at first, you swell up with gas, belch and become constipated.

The Secret of Bushman's Digestive Advantage

I returned to school in my forties in Chicago to study chiropractic medicine. During my private investigations after class I read Rasmussen's "The Hypophysis Cerebri (the pituitary gland) of Bushman, the Gorilla of Lincoln Park Zoo, Chicago."[7] For years thereafter, I continued visiting the zoo on most weekends, as I had done from my teens when I studied dentistry at Northwestern University, and analyzed Bushman during his feeding periods. Space forbids my going into detail of how I detected psychically, odically and physiologically, through my psychic power center and through visual observation, the unsuspected effects of Bushman's not-so-rudimentary intermediate lobe on his digestion. I realized that I had made one of the foremost and most practical miracle discoveries of all times.

How I Transferred the Secret of Bushman's Extraordinary Digestive Power Into My Own Digestion

I concluded that it would take too long to rejuvenate the intermediate lobe of my (or your) pituitary gland. I determined, instead, to find out how to *trigger the effects* of such a miraculous rejuvenation of my digestion on me. After several months of self-experimentation I found the method. I had to project the odic force of my intermediate lobe downwards into my intestines and forcibly implant the odic force of the food I was digesting into the walls of my intestines. To my feverish delight, it worked!

It was the birth of the Triple Tonic Secret. Swiftly, I devised an easy way to bring it about by dividing the process into three simple steps:

1. I visualized my food being masticated and its specific nutrients being digested normally. (Illus. 5A).
2. I visualized my food being absorbed in my intestines, but its odic force not being pressed into intimate contact with my intestinal wall (which contains my intestinal muscles). (Illus. 5B).
3. I then blasted the full power of the odic force of my intermediate lobe upon the odic force of the food and implanted both into my intestinal wall. (Illus. 5C). Driving it from high in my head to my abdomen, I could drill the odic force of my pituitary down into my intestinal wall with miraculous psychic leverage.

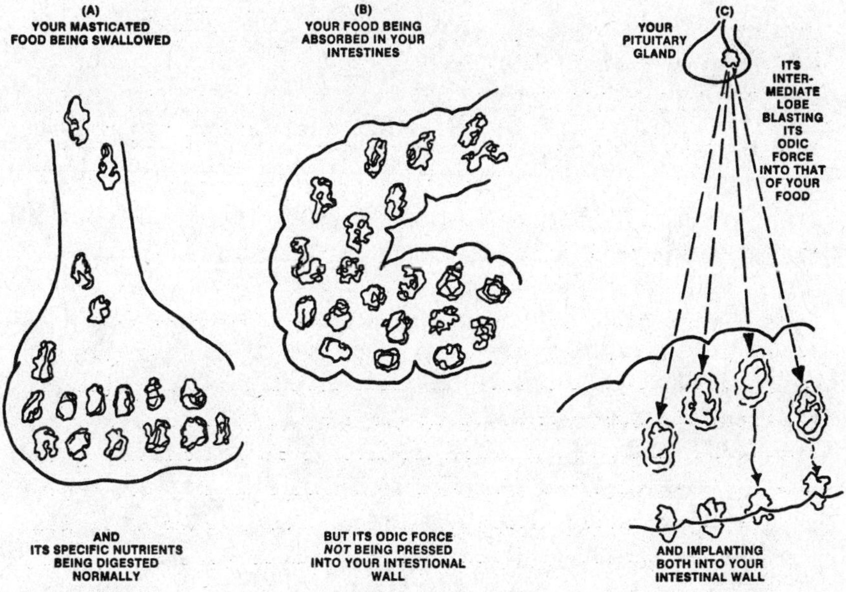

Illustration 5

That is the Triple Tonic Secret. My digestion improved as if by magic. I felt twenty years younger and my waist shrank. Although I was making no effort to fast or starve, my appetite was satisfied more swiftly now because my tissues were *more* completely "nutrified" with less food. I have taught the Triple Tonic Secret to hundreds of people since, and they call it a miracle. In *Solar Diet* I revealed to my readers the *record way* to lose weight without pills, special diet or surgery, as the *record natural way* to lose weight. I am revealing to you now, as part of *Yogatronics*, the Triple Tonic Secret to improve on that record, thereby keeping my dietary discoveries *another 23 years* ahead of science.. Project it to your food every time you eat.

The New Mental You Resulting from the Triple Tonic Secret

I urge you, hereafter, to fall in love with your own waist, the axis of your whole body! Turn physiologically narcissistic! Embrace total health and long-lasting youth as your constant mistress or lover! Explode with ecstasy from your waistline and ring with muscle tone. Cast out flabby relaxation from your whole body, and the negativity of mental suppression. Thunder forth irresistibly, as Don Quixote tried to do, although he lacked the magic odic force of the hard small waist to achieve his dreams. Don't collapse into a physiological nonentity, but vibrate and conquer! Make your every wish come true with the mind-body lightness that makes you feel, act and look like someone half your age. I did it. Join me and do it, too!

What Yogatronics Will Do for You

To possess a youthful, trim and healthy waist, you require a trim and healthy body. You even require a healthy-looking skin, for instance, for a "bad" skin robs you of self-confidence and fills you with stress. The next chapters show you the easy permanent way to acquire a youthful trim body and a small waist and how to prevent any other part of your body from sabotaging your efforts. They teach you how to reach your peak in health, the feeling of youth, looking much younger, mental keenness, psychic power, sex appeal, money-making capacity, excellence at sports, beauty of body, impressiveness of physique, physical endurance, limitless energy without pills or drugs or special diet and—lastt but not least—how to be wasp-waisted for the rest of your life. Also, they show you how to achieve all these goals in the swiftest, healthiest and simplest way imaginable. You can do it all, besides, probably 23 *years* before science knows the method.

REFERENCES

[1]*Zodic Force Control: Secret of Miracle Healing and Long Life*, (Parker Publishing Company, Inc., West Nyack, N.Y. 1977)

[2]*Chicago Tribune*, August 14, 1977.

[3]Dr. I. Sukharbsky, director of the Public Institute of Juvinolog, and L. V. Romanov, biologist at the Institute of General Genetics and vice-chairman of a newly formed National Committee on the Artificial Prolongation of Human Life. *Los Angeles Times*, August, 1977.

[4]A. T. Rassmussen 1936. "The Proportions of the Various Subdivisions of the Normal Adult Human Hypophysis Cerebri," etc. In: *Research Nerv. and Ment. Dis., The Pituitary Gland.* Williams & Wilkins, Baltimore. 118-150.

[5]William Boyd, M.D., *A Text Book of Pathology, An Introduction to Medicine*, Sixth Edition. (Lea & Febiger, Philadelphia, 1953, p. 727).

[6]Harvey Ernest Jordan, *A Textbook of Histology*, Ninth Edition. (Appleton-Century-Crofts, Inc., New York, 1952), p. 202.

[7]A. T. Rasmussen, and T. Rasmussen. 1952. "The Hypophysis Cerebri of Bushman, the Gorilla of Lincoln Park Zoo." Chicago, *Anat. Rec.*, *113*, 325-347.

3

Yogatronics: The Magic Road to a Streamlined Body and Youthful Skin

How a Fine Skin Controls Your Trimness and Small Waist

Without a fine skin, as stated before, you won't have a trim figure and a small waist. An "unwise" diet plagues your skin with blemishes, dryness or oiliness, unnecessary wrinkles, areas of pigmentation and an aging, leathery texture. It also constipates you, threatens your stomach and liver, acidifies your blood, dulls your mentality, weakens your muscles, depletes your endurance and ruins your teeth. It reduces your energy and activity and accumulates unwanted fat and cholesterol deposits in your organs and arteries. To avoid such a diet, a prominent California nutrition consultant, Miss Irene Holbrook of Santa Monica, offered rules to keep the skin beautiful through good nutrition. They turned out to be *identical* with the diet rules I published in *Solar Diet* 23 years before. But the *Yogatronic Diet* goes even deeper into these rules and adds the 9th Magic Rule to them. Read them below and apply them.

Rule 1. *What Kind of Foods to Consume.* For a good skin, the prominent nutritionist recommends consuming *many fiber foods.*

The *Yogatronic Diet* goes even deeper than that. *Yogatronics* declares that chronic and persistent attacks of pimples can result from an overacid diet. From such a diet, your skin turns sallow, the whites of your eyes turn yellow and your whole body and brain become lethargic. Overacidity is something to guard against if you want to live a long, healthy life and look young until the very last. Most fresh fruits and vegetables are alkaline, because they oxidize into alkalis during the process of digestion. Fresh fruits and vegetables are fiber foods.

Fiber foods, by filling you sooner, also satisfy your appetite sooner and lessen the amount of calories you consume. They thereby limit the amount of fat your body is likely to add whenever you eat. They reduce your weight, too, by holding water, easing your evacuations and emptying your body of more wastes when your bowels move. They excrete more of the fats of food from your body. All these features, together, reduce your waist and your whole body.

Rule 2. *What to Drink—and How Much.* For a good skin the nutritionist recommends *drinking a lot of water.* Not necessarily eight glasses a day, she explained, but that amount would help to wash out the "metabolic by-products" that brought on your skin problems.

Yogatronics goes even deeper than that. The first thing to take when you get up in the morning is a glass of warm water with the juice of half a lemon. To save your teeth from erosion, suck it up through a straw and swallow it immediately. Then rinse your mouth. This drink soothes your stomach, neutralizes its acidity and fills you with appetite. When your stomach is acid, your appetite decreases. When it is alkaline, your appetite increases. Between breakfast and lunch, drink three or four glasses of water. Have another glass or two about 1 to 1-1/2 hours after breakfast. Have another glass or two about 1 to 1-1/4 hours after that. Drink *nothing* for an hour before lunch. You *should* drink several glasses of water between lunch and supper. Take only a glass of water between supper and bedtime. More than that may keep you getting up in the night, and less than that lets your stomach stay too acid after supper. Neither eat nor drink before going to bed. Don't even drink a fruit or vegetable juice. That certainly amounts to drinking "plenty of water," as the prominent nutritionist advises, totaling about 8 glasses.

This water, plus that in your breakfast food, will drive you to the lavatory about twice during the morning. This is only natural, so don't be alarmed. Water between meals also keeps your digesting food irrigated. This helps to discourage it from forming hard, compact, severely constipating masses. It helps to keep your colon moist and soft—not dry and hard. It helps to keep your blood from turning too acid or from retaining the metabolic by-products that can bring on skin problems, as it is likely to do after a heavy energizing meal.

Drinking lots of water, therefore, has much the same effect as fiber foods in keeping your bowels moving easier, thus reducing the size of your waist and maintaining your whole body youthful and trim. It protects your skin from turning dry, leathery and old-looking. It diminishes your calorie intake by filling your stomach enough between meals to discourage you from eating snacks, which would automatically add to your weight and to the girth of your waist. Temporarily, fibrous foods produce more gas in your lower intestines and distend your waist. But your fecal matter will be more solid and move more slowly otherwise and "permanently" bulge at your waist until you eliminate it with enemas, laxatives or other unnatural means. By drinking enough water between meals you lessen that accumulation of gas and regain a trim, flat-waisted look.

Rule 3. *Foods to Stop Eating.* For a good skin, the nutritionist recommends you stop eating cane sugar and refined flour products. These, she explains, contain empty calories and little or no protein, vitamins or minerals.

Yogatronics explores this more thoroughly. Sugar is acid, or—through chemical reaction—turns your stomach acid. A candy bar eaten before your meal will ruin your appetite. You feel full, but you are actually starving. Keep away from highly refined, degerminized cereals. Such "softened" cereals sometimes have their valuable elements removed, and they can turn "concrete-like" in your intestines, blow you up with gas and ruin the flatness of your abdomen. They can severely constipate you, because they have been deprived of their roughage. *Roughage* foods pass through you readily. They are too bulky to be compressed into tightly packed, dry masses. Their bulk, too, tends to stimulate bowel action. When you like sweets too much, you also dislike vegetables, fresh fruits and fresh meat. You become a chronic dyspeptic, acquire a wretched complexion, and suffer from vitamin starvation.

Let me add that Claude Bernard (1813-1878) found that your blood loses about one third of the sugar it carries while streaming from your arteries to your veins. It leaves one third of its sugar behind for your tissues to use. I contend that when it leaves more than that behind in your tissues or more sugar than your muscles use for energy, the extra amount, is deposited in your skin, where your capillaries empty. Since your capillary blood contains one-fourth more sugar than your venous blood, sugar is left behind in your skin, more so in certain spots than others. Being a foreign matter, this excess sugar irritates these spots in your skin and creates an area of inflammation, or a pimple.

Rule 4. *Other Drinks and Foods and a Beautiful Skin.* If you imbibe alcoholic beverages, the well-known nutritionist recommends that you do so only moderately. Such an addiction could curse your skin with a puffy look and make you appear older than you are.

Yogatronics discloses still more. The *Yogatronic Diet* recommends *no liquor.* Liquor of any kind is a stomach acidifier. Beer and wine not only turn it acid but put on fat-weight. When they retain fluids in your body, they certainly put on "fat-weight." Harsher liquors, like whiskey, should be avoided completely.

Rule 5. *Vitamins and Minerals for Good Skin.* The nutritionist recommends food high in vitamins and minerals but not in fat and sugar, to maintain good skin.

Yogatronics adds a word about cereal. If your problem is excess weight, you had better leave out the cereal altogether, or just take a spoonful of it. Supplant it with sea food tablets. They are very low in calories and high in energy value. The sea plants are rich natural sources of thirty-eight minerals and trace minerals.

Rule 6. *Whole Grain Food for Fine Skin.* For a good skin, the nutritionist recommends eating two servings of whole grain daily.

Yogatronics brings still more to light. Cereal whole grain or meat makes a fine, heavy, sustaining breakfast food. Meat, if not fried or heavily seasoned, does not add to your weight and is more easily digested than cereal. If you are inclined to be *underweight*, eat breakfast cereal from four to five times a week. Eat bread only once a day. Cereal, in the morning, is all the grain you need at that time.

Rule 7. *Protein Makes for Healthy Skin.* The nutritionist recommends at least two servings of protein food a day for a good skin.

Yogatronics elucidates further. To prepare the meat, broil, bake or stew it. A very good breakfast meat is liver, briefly simmered in a small amount of water. However, liver, being an organ meat, is flooded with man-made chemicals. For suppers, the so-called "red" meats (lean beef, veal, mutton, lamb) are very good. Chicken, duck and other game birds are good food, too, although they don't build up your blood or your muscles like animal meat. But, unless they are too fat, they are easy to digest. That makes two servings of protein food.

Rule 8. *The Magic Salad for Attractive Skin.* For a good skin, Miss Holbrook recommends two or more servings of green, leafy vegetables a day.

Yogatronics expounds beyond that. An excellent breakfast dish is a big plate of a favorite fruit or a fresh salad bowl. Also start your supper with a lighter plate, like a salad. Never skip the salad for supper. All meals should start off with lighter food, then proceed to heavier foods and climax with a beverage. Since the heavier food digests more slowly, eat it last so it won't slow down the digestion of the lighter food and cause it to putrify in your stomach. The supper salad is a great revitalizer and alkalizer. Your salad should consist of *raw* vegetables without unhealthy seasonings. It should consist of leafy vegetables like lettuce, endive, watercress, escarole and of solid, bulky vegetables like carrots, beets, parsnips and celery (the green variety, not the bleached). Do not masticate these solid vegetables, or they will grind down your teeth. Use a food shredder or grater. Don't try to soften these foods by cooking—no matter how little. The only necessary exceptions to this rule are such vegetables as winter squash, string beans and, possibly, potatoes. These should be baked or cooked by some waterless method. Next best would be to boil them in their well-scrubbed jackets and use the potato water in soup to save the minerals. Remember, all forms of cooking destroy some of the vitamins and minerals in vegetables, as well as reduce their constipation-relieving bulk. Enough vitamins are lost by storage in the refrigerator and by the necessary scrubbing with brush and mild soap before they are grated. Give them a thorough quick rinsing. Don't let them soak in the water, but be sure to rinse *all* the soap off them. Place the lettuce in the salad bowl, then the shredded or grated vegetables on top of the lettuce and make the dish tasty by slicing or cubing a fresh tomato into it.

More Magic Salad for Attractive Skin

A serving spoon of home-baked beans on top of the salad bowl makes an appetizing variation. Beans have lately been found to be a most effective preventer of cholesterol deposits in the body. Above all, don't wreck your salad with any of the salad dressings composed of condiments, vinegar and oil. If you do not put on weight easily, a few drops of vegetable, peanut or olive oil can be added to your salad to make it tasty. But remember, the salad's tastelessness is its healthy alkalinity. Condiments, spices and vinegar fill your stomach with acid. Vinegar also erodes your teeth while in your mouth, and since the oils require so much longer to digest than the salad, I advise you to add no oil to your salad. The oil will coat your salad and prevent it from being digested in your stomach. Your salad will have to wait for several hours to reach your intestines, to be digested only *after* covering oil is digested. By then, it will be putrefied. Anyway, your intestines contain no enzymes to digest your salad. A considerable portion of your salad passes through your stools undigested and leave you bloated with gas, when you cover it with oil.

Raw onion, sliced very thin, also adds taste to your salad. Onions also help purify your blood and lower your cholesterol level.

Warning About Preparing the Salad. When you prepare the salad, don't ruin its food value by over tampering with it before serving it. Plan your meal preparation so that the salad is prepared just before it is eaten. The moment live food is cut and exposed to air, its vitamin and mineral content deplete fast. Do not let your fresh raw food stand around for too long after it is cut and ready to eat. Keep it covered tightly, too, meanwhile, to protect it from light and air. Both of these destroy important vitamins with alarming rapidity.

Rule 9. *Magic Fruit for Colorful Skin.* For good skin, the nutritionist recommends two or more servings of fruit a day.

Yogatronics reveals still more by maintaining that a good breakfast should consist of a light, liquid food (like a fruit); a heavier food (like a salad or cereal) to fill you and stay with you, a predominantly bowel-moving food (like prunes) and a warming, energizing finisher (like warm milk). A breakfast consisting of more or less than that is not the kind of breakfast that *Yogatronics* recommends. The *Yogatronic Diet* suggests eating "a light liquid food" (like fruit) at lunch time, but to eat a big, fibrous salad at breakfast because it will stay with you better until lunch.

An ideal staying-with-you lunch fruit is the banana. It is still a fruit, thus it is comparatively easy to digest. But, it is also heavy enough to stay with you for hours after your meal. It won't constipate you, like the usual sandwich, but neither will it encourage loose bowels. It builds up your body weight, too, but does not fatten. And it is available most of the year.

Supper Fruit for Colorful Skin

Fresh pineapple, watermelon, apples, grapefruit, oranges, tomatoes, are great mucus-killing foods to eat at supper.

That constitutes three servings of fruit a day, and again fits "the Beautiful Skin Diet" of this prominent nutritionist. Mucous-forming foods leave you easily fatigued, and so you become less active and gain unnecessary weight. Mucous-forming foods also turn your body acid, which, as I stated earlier, ruins your skin. They leave you more susceptible to colds. Illness reduces your energy and activity, which in turn adds to the size of your waist.

Rule 10. *The Magic Beverage for Clear Skin.* Miss Holbrook recommends drinking two glasses of skim milk a day for a good skin.

Yogatronics maintains that your breakfast is not complete without the warm, energizing finisher. Coffee, tea or chocolate are too acid-creating for that. Milk, warmed to a degree, is better. It is a natural food and contains valuable food elements, even if it loses many of them during pasteurization. If overweight is your problem, don't eliminate milk from your diet. Skim milk contains everything in whole milk, except the fattening butterfat. Both liquid and dry, milk solids are now available in most food stores.

The supper beverage should be much like the breakfast beverage. Milk is a fine supper beverage, because it stays with you. Certain people, it is believed, do not digest milk because they lack the enzyme which digests the galactose sugar in the milk. I personally believe that anybody can digest milk—particularly skim milk—if he drinks it slowly and does not exercise, bend over or engage in unusual physical activity for two hours afterwards. Still, I don't dispute the laboratory conclusion. You can always try a more easily digestible milk, like buttermilk or yogurt. Otherwise, shift to fruit or vegetable juices. Milk, though, is a required food for a beautiful skin because of its ample content of vitamin A. For your waist and weight, raw whole milk contains too much fat and will enlarge both of them. Skim milk will keep them trim and will not slow down your bowels. Buttermilk or yogurt, of course, will reduce both your weight and your waist. But they might reduce you so much that they leave your face drawn. Perhaps you can take less of them if that happens. If your face is naturally fleshy or round and doesn't look drawn easily, you need not worry. A thin drawn face makes anyone look older than he is, even though some faces are naturally thin and drawn; but constipation, bloated abdomen, indigestion or too slow digestion will also cause your face to look thinner and drawn and detract from the appearance of your skin. It helps your skin when you control the size of your waist by following the *Yogatronic Diet*, whose basic tenets were set down in *Solar Diet* 23 years before a prominent nutritionist upheld them, practically to the letter.

Diet Secrets for a Rosy Complexion

When your diet lacks enough fat, your skin suffers. When you become discouraged you are prone to let yourself get heavier and bigger around the waist. If you add foods containing linoleic, linolenic and arachidonic fatty acids to your diet, your skin will improve surprisingly. You can then regain your enthusiasm, take better care of yourself again and trim down your body and your waist. These fatty acids are essential. Vitamin B_6 also helps. Eat bananas, beef kidney, dry skim milk, whole rice, soybeans, dry brewer's yeast and wheat germ. (*Note*: I have never taken any kind of yeast).

Your skin will turn dry and scaly if you don't eat enough vitamin A. Your hair follicles change, and your oil and sweat glands dry up. The best sources of vitamin A are cod-liver oil and other fish-liver oils. Possibly excepting cod-liver oil, I recommend no oils in concentrated form, because they are hard to digest. Such oils seem to bloat the waist and overwork the stomach and liver. Other good sources of vitamin A which seem easy to digest are fish roe, the flesh of oily fish, the livers of other animals (although livers nowadays are the filtering plants of man-made chemicals), butter, eggs and cheese. The pro-vitamins (vitamin-makers) of vitamin A are found abundantly in carrots and other yellow vegetables, like squash and sweet potatoes, and in many green vegetables, particularly broccoli, spinach and beet greens. (Spinach and beet greens, though, contain considerable oxalic acid, which can accumulate in your kidneys and form kidney stones). No food, however, compares to beets for giving you a rosy complexion. Yellow maize, escarole, water cress, string beans, green peas, pumpkin, bananas and cantaloupe are also rich in vitamin A. It is stored mainly in your liver (95 percent), but also in the cortex of your adrenal glands, your retina, your corpus luteum (woman) and body fat. To have a good supply of it in your body you need a good liver. To help you acquire one, do *The Abdominal Double Curl*. (Illus. 6). *Note:* If you take cod-liver oil, take the normal doses set forth on the bottle, unless you take it under prescription. Mix it in ⅓d of a cup of skim milk. Take it at the end of breakfast and supper, as a food, not as a medicine.

THE ABDOMINAL DOUBLE CURL—TO REDUCE YOUR BODY SAG—AND RESTORE YOUR NATURAL, INBORN SEX VIGOR

The position to assume

1. Lie flat on your bed, or on a softened floor. Do not lie on the hard, bare floor.

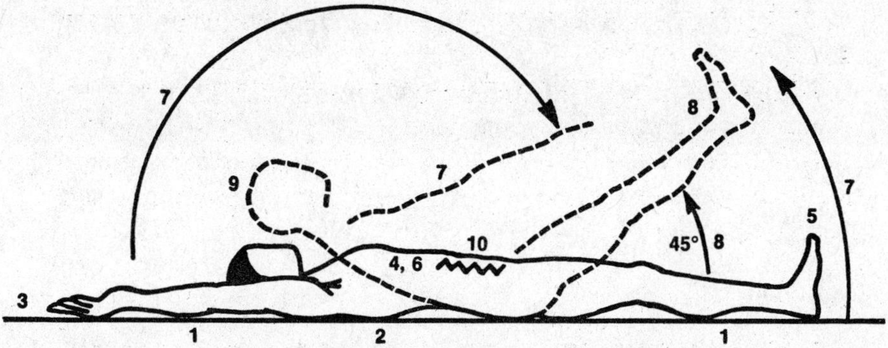

Illustration 6

2. Lie on your back.
3. Stretch arms out directly in back of your head.

How to do this simple movement

4. Inhale deeply.
5. Curl your toes towards your head.
6. Now, gather your strength and *exhale* as you
7. Raise your arms and legs at the same time.
8. Raise your legs no higher than 45 degrees from the ground.
9. Raise your body as you bring your arms forwards and downwards, as if trying to touch your toes with your fingers.
10. Relax and repeat.

This simple movement develops:

1. Rectus abdominis. (The horizontal grooves across the front of your waist.)
2. External and internal obliques (the muscles of the fronts and sides of your waist).

Frequency

20-200 times a day, in groups of 10 repetitions.

This is perhaps the greatest abdominal "shrinker" of them all. It is hard to do, but it works miracles for your waistline, stomach, circulation and heart, for it makes it beat fast almost immediately. Making your heart beat fast once a day is one sure way to keep the fat off it.

Make this simple movement a regular routine for the rest of your life.*

Eliminate cane sugar to have a small waist and normal weight, because you ought to keep your blood sugar as normal as possible. You won't use up enough of the sugar in your food otherwise, and your body will store the excess in your liver and in your skin, causing pimples.

Foods Your Skin Needs

With respect to the essential fatty acids which your skin needs, some people need more than others. You will find these essential fatty acids in cod-liver oil, butter (very small amounts), linseed oil, halibut oil, olive oil, peanut oil, soybean oil and many other oils. However, I caution you once more against taking oils if they "bother" your digestion. I prefer raw peanuts and soybeans to their oils. The only essential fatty acid you miss then is found mostly in lard, but I don't recommend lard because of its heavy concentration of artery-narrowing saturated fat. Don't eat rancid fats. They nullify the benefits of vitamins A and E. And, while the outer leaves of lettuce contain 30 times more vitamin A (or its provitamin) than the inner white leaves, they also contain far more insecticide spray.

All the B-vitamins are removed from refined foods and are replaced only partially with synthetic vitamins. These include essential vitamins, like choline (which removes fat), and pyridoxine. (Pyridoxine helps to metabolize the fats and the *essential* fatty acids you eat.) In its absence, you metabolize *undesirable* fatty acids, add weight and enlarge your waistline. The B vitamins also include inositol, which prevents your stomach from emptying too fast, before it has absorbed enough nourishment out of your food. B-vitamins rank among your most important food needs.

Avoid chocolate and cocoa. They fatten you, constipate you and round out your waist. I have repeatedly accused chocolate of wrecking the skin, and both chocolate and cocoa acidify the stomach and the blood. Both are rich in calcium, but also contain oxalic acid. Oxalic acid renders their calcium unavailable to the body and robs it of the calcium it has already stored.

*Reprinted from YOGA FOR MEN ONLY. Dr. Frank Rudolph Young, 1968. With permission.

The Condemned Food that Beautifies Your Skin

Eat foods with lecithin to help ward off unwanted disfigurements on your skin like: horny growths, pigmented patches, a bronzing of your skin (indication of fat deficiency), senile shrinking of your skin, greasy skin and even pimples. Egg yolks are probably the best source of lecithin. I have eaten eggs my whole life, and my heart and circulation are in great shape. Although egg yolks are condemned for their alarming content of cholesterol, the lecithin in the egg yolk apparently nullifies the effects of the cholesterol in it. As I revealed in my long interview for the *Chicago Tribune* (conducted by Jeff Lyon for his Close Up column), I exercise vigorously 3 to 4 hours a day with my private disciple, William Adams Lowry. And, five nights a week, before going to bed at the end of my 10-hour working day plus my 4 hours of exercise, I perform an incredible feat of heart power. I run up twelve flights of steep, indoor fire-escape stairs at top speed by two's, without stopping or coasting along the way. A minute and a half later, however, my heart is beating normally again and I feel totally refreshed. To judge from a table of energy expenditure per hour, that exertion uses up about five times the energy of "strenuous exercise."

And I eat eggs every day! In my late teens and early twenties I ate six a day, but my impoverished state later on compelled me to reduce them to two a day. I still eat from one to two a day, at breakfast. I heat water to a boil, turn off the stove and drop the eggs into the water for about two-and-a-half minutes. I never salt them, but eat them at the end of breakfast because the fat in the yolk digests more slowly than the other food.

The American Journal of Chemical Nutrition, May, 1977, reveals that three separate studies in Sofia, Prague and Illinois prove that "eggs do not raise cholesterol levels." Volunteers ate 2 eggs a day *over and above* their usual diets. Four hours later there was *no* change in the blood cholesterol levels "in the majority of patients." The majority proves the rule.

How Sally K. Lost 20 Lbs. and Her Sallow Complexion

At first sight people thought that Sally K. had liver trouble because her complexion was so sallow. She was 20 pounds overweight, was very attractive in conversation and a most satisfactory worker. But she was unusually sensitive about her appearance because it detracted from her appeal. Her health was satisfactory, but her employer watched her changing figure and her sallow complexion with suspicion.

With the *Yogatronic Diet* Sally's bowels started moving regularly. Bananas, beef kidney, dry skim milk, whole rice, soybeans, beets and wheat germ restored her rosy complexion. She lost her extra 20 lbs., and her figure changed unbelievably. She soon had a steady boyfriend. Every time she ate, she projected the Triple Tonic secret within her and into her food.

How Tina U. Lost Her Unwanted Bulk and Her Dried-Up Look

Tina U. dreaded to see herself in the mirror. Lines she had never expected to acquire were forming on her face while she was still young. She had skipped the fun in life to get where she was, but the youth-look was deserting her fast. She lost interest in her future and gained more weight. She took different oils for her skin, but they disturbed her digestion.

The *Yogatronic Diet* automatically supplied her with other natural, but not concentrated, sources of vitamin A, such as the flesh of oily fish, carrots and other yellow vegetables like squash and green vegetables like broccoli. She stayed away from refined foods but ate one egg a day. Every time she ate, she projected the Tonic secret within her and into her food.

Tina's skin turned smoother by the day. She lost weight and her waist shrank. In a few weeks she looked so comparatively young and enthusiastic that she attracted the very man she wanted most, who had ignored her before. Life, she sighed, had *not* passed her by.

4

Stay Young the Yogatronics Way—By Keeping Your Insides Slim

The Primary Way to Keep Down Waist-Swelling Gas

Digestive diseases are the nation's third largest killer, but they are the most neglected affliction in America. More people suffer from digestive disorders than from heart disease. Funds for research in them, nonetheless, are very short, and medical authorities have pointed out that most doctors don't receive enough training in them. Unless you keep your digestion at its best, you cannot expect to maintain your ideal weight or waist size. Your stomach and intestines will bloat and drag your rib-box down upon your abdomen and bulge it even more. Your bowels will either move too much or too little or retain wastes in you that fatigue you and reduce your activity or exercise. You will be saddled with still more weight and "permanently" retained gas. Fat, too, will accummulate around your liver, stomach, intestines, heart and kidneys.

Eating salted snack foods (eating any snack food) on an empty stomach can balloon it by stimulating it to secrete an excess of hydrochloric acid. The excess salt, through osmosis, draws excess liquid out of your bloodstream through your stomach walls into your stomach and causes you to belch as your stomach blows up abnormally. Its stretched nerves shoot sensations of pain to your brain and can annoy you with headaches and crawling sensations. Alkaline foods, like pineapple and papaya, help reduce such bulging by neutralizing the excess hydrochloric acid in your stomach, but soybeans and other legumes counteract the alkalizing effects of these fruits because they inhibit their trypsin-like enzymes.

What Alcohol Can do to Your Body and Waist

Alcohol increases the amount of hydrochloric acid your stomach secretes and increases its acidity. This produces gas and bloating and a low-grade gastritis (inflammation of your stomach). Alcohol simultaneously decreases the amount of protein-digesting enzyme that your stomach secretes. That causes the protein you eat to putrefy in your stomach instead of being digested, and distends it with gas. Alcohol also robs your body of vitamin B_1, enlarges your heart, diminishes your vital capacity and creates lesions in your heart. Recent research, true enough, shows that people who drink several glasses of beer a day, die less often of heart disease than those who don't. But it ignores the evidence that drinkers eat less than non-drinkers because alcohol diminishes their appetites, perhaps because of the low-grade gastritis with which alcohol afflicts them at first. The undisciplined non-drinker, in contrast, can consume food with too much cholesterol because he can digest it easier than the drinker. The excess cholesterol invades his arteries and his heart. The *drinker*, with his decreased appetite will therefore consume far less high-cholesterol food than the teetotaler.

But the teetotaler does not *have* to eat foods high in cholesterol. He can stop doing that easily with the *Yogatronic Diet*, as you will see. But the drinker's waist will bulge more and more as his liver turns fibrous (cirrhosis) and the gas in his stomach rounds it out still more. He will have less energy to be active, exercise and tone up his abdominal muscles because he will be ill-nourished.

How Other Foods Hold Down the Size of Your Waist

You need folic acid to maintain the normal food absorption of your stomach and intestines. Part of your food, otherwise, will pass through your alimentary canal unabsorbed and produce gas, discomfort, headaches, constipation, lassitude and an appetite for health-wrecking foods. It will make you heavier and enlarge your waist. Good sources of folic acid are yeast, cauliflower, liver and kidney (although the last two are organ meats, and they are saturated with man-made chemicals added to the soil and to the animal's body by injection). Fair sources of folic acid are beef, veal and wheat. Poor sources are root vegetables, tomatoes, bananas, rice, corn, sweet potatoes, pork, ham and lamb. Folic acid has some relationship to vitamin C. Since alcohol causes a vitamin C deficiency, it also causes a folic acid deficiency and lessens the food absorption in your stomach and intestines.

Eggs help your digestion because their lecithin increases the digestibility and absorption of the fats in your food.

Gastrointestinal disturbances caused by alcohol and hard-to-digest foods, like fried or highly spiced dishes, decrease your normal absorption of iron from your food and impoverish your blood and the hemoglobin content of its red blood cells. The amount of oxygen your tissues absorb when you exercise or engage in everyday activity will be reduced and you will fatigue sooner. But, your appetite will not diminish and you will gain weight and a bigger waist.

How Losing Some Weight Can Mislead You

Your liver, like your kidneys, stomach and intestines, does not "age." All these organs are structured to last at least 150 years. They can last twice as long if you take as fine care of them as you do of your car or your lawn. Your liver's ability to clear poisons from your body lessens with extreme old age, but it possesses such stupendous built-in reserves that it can still do a satisfactory job. After all, you don't get jaundiced naturally as you grow old.

When you abuse your liver from childhood up, by overconsuming sugar and sugar products, you subject it to a savage ordeal. Even your best foods, today, contain enough toxic substances to punish your liver mercilessly and convert large numbers of its normal cells into non-functioning fibrous (cirrhotic) cells. Men are mainly affected by cirrhosis in late-middle life, although women are catching up to them. By then, your liver is practically butchered. Your food seldom digests "right," even though, after diagnosis, "nothing" may be found wrong with you and you think you have a "nervous" stomach. Frequently, your appetite deserts you, particularly for nutritious food. You are plagued with annoying gas, slight dizziness, even with a fleeting tenderness on the right side of your abdomen. And, you lose weight.

Losing weight, however, does not necessarily indicate that your waistline is smaller. It may be bigger, in fact, or appear bigger because your chest sinks downwards from the resulting fatigue and listlessness. You become more inactive, more of your muscle cells degenerate into fat and increase your total "fat-weight." Yet, you might weigh less on the scales. An alarming proportion of this "fat-weight," besides, might line the insides of your arteries with cholesterol plaques, infiltrate your heart, liver, kidneys, adrenal glands and other cholesterol depots. But you stop worrying—because you *weigh* less. You weigh less only because your muscles have softened and lost bulk. But you have gained *deadly* "fat-weight." To your consternation, you probably measure more now around your flabby waist, although you may weigh many pounds less.

Your Hidden Liver Ruiner

You may be consuming far more sugar than you dream. Sugar is hidden in much of your processed food and prepared food. Your liver is repeatedly flooded with excess glucose. It can hold no more than 150 grams of glycogen (stored sugar, ready for use by your muscles or for body energy, when needed), so it transforms the excess into fat globules. If you are a man they are deposited primarily over your abdomen, the sides of your waist, and under your chin. If you are a woman they are also deposited on your thighs, breasts, neck, back, hips, and backs of your upper arms. Because of the abuse you are inflicting on your liver, "strain hollows" encircle your eyes, and you feel as if you are recovering from a hang-over. There is no need to explain the damage being done to your teeth and bones by their being robbed of calcium and necessary vitamins. Just remember that "cheap" sugar is 99.5 percent carbohydrate. It contains no calcium, phosphorus or vitamins. White sugar does not nourish you at all because its vitamins have been removed in the refinement process. That includes candy, cakes, soft drinks, chewing gum and jelly sandwiches. Eating them between meals eventually ruins your digestion.

Diet Secrets to Limit the Acidity of Your Blood and Urine

Most of your body fluids are alkaline. Your urine may be acidic, and your gastric juice is very acidic, but those are the exceptions. When you don't eat enough protein, or when you eat so much sugar or fat that you lose your appetite for less tasty but more nutritious food, the protein content of your blood plasma falls to a low. This also happens when you exercise so soon after a meal that your liver can't function properly. Your kidneys are overburdened by the excess of sugar and eliminate it into your urine, but you are wearing out your kidneys and accumulating excess acid in your system. You become constipated and lose your physical vigor. You feel like being less active and exercising less. You start getting fat, and your waist enlarges. Your bladder is irritated by the excess sugar passing out of you and is headed for trouble. Your intestines could be developing ulcers.

The proteins (and nucleoproteins) you eat break down in your body to form, among other chemical compounds, sulfuric and other acids. The fruits and vegetables you eat, with their calcium, magnesium, sodium and potassium, usually combine with the acids produced by the proteins you eat and lessen the acidity in your blood and urine. If not for this combination, you would develop the serious condition of acidosis, and your kidneys and bladder would be ruined with Bright's disease and inflammation of your bladder (cystitis). Citric acid (present in oranges, grapefruits, lemon), malic acid (in apples), and lactic acid (in milk) help you by oxidizing your "protein acids." That's why vegetables and acid fruits (including pineapple) usually have an alkaline effect on your body. Citrus fruits are ingested as acid, but their metals form alkaline compounds and alkalize your bloodstream.

Exceptions Among Foods—Which Keep Your Blood and Urine Acid

Benzoic acid (found in cranberries) is an exception and does not alkalize your bloodstream. It is not oxidized by your body but is excreted as hippuric acid, which increases the acidity of your urine. Another exception is oxalic acid. It is found in beet leaves, chocolate, cocoa, tea, prunes, plums, rhubarb, spinach. It is found in small amounts in potatoes, beans, root beets, tomatoes, cauliflower, onions, mushrooms, celery, currants, raspberries, grapes and pears. Spinach and rhubarb contain an extraordinary amount of it, making them inadvisable to eat. Oxalic acid combines with the acid in your blood to form crystals of calcium oxalate. These crystals are deposited in your kidneys and form a large part of most kidney stones and gallstones. It is risky to consume large servings of rhubarb over an extended period of time. Even if rhubarb contains a lot of calcium, other foods contain as much calcium with less oxalic acid. Among these are lettuce, broccoli, dandelion, loose leaf cabbage, Brussel sprouts, kohlrabi, collards, turnip greens, watercress, mustard greens, and others. These foods won't form stones in your kidneys and gall bladder.

But, there is a dangerous source of oxalic acid which you may not suspect. It can be triggered by exercising too soon after eating meat or sugar or by eating too much of either at one time so that they slow down your digestion and putrefy in your digestive tract. Meat and sugar are free of oxalic acid. But, when they are thrown into a state of extreme fermentation, they can cause marked oxalic poisoning in your body and strain your kidneys.

Why I have Persistently Opposed High-Protein Diets

I have opposed high-protein diets from the time of their inception, as far back as 1952 when I advised the young weight-lifter and body builder, who soon won all the top physique titles including Mr. Universe, to stop using such pills. With them, he developed his muscles larger than ever and reduced the size of his waist to a washboard look. I opposed the pills because the more protein you take beyond your daily requirement, the more urea and uric acid it produces for your kidneys to eliminate. Twenty-five years later, a number of healthy women between 25 and 44 died while taking liquid protein on a diet to reduce weight. Their hearts seemed to stop beating because of an extraordinary loss of potassium. Too much urea and uric acid in the urine cause the bloodstream to use up an abnormally large quantity of potassium carbonate to neutralize it and maintain the acid-base balance. So, my warning to him, even though I could not explain it scientifically at the time, was astute. Twenty-five years later science reveals the reason. The *Yogatronic Diet* does not produce a potassium imbalance in the body and thus helps to prolong life instead of shortening it. That's how it helps to keep your insides slim, your body trim and your waist small. *And it does so in a safe, healthy fashion!*

Illustration 7 teaches you the Triple Tonic Secret to increase the effectiveness of your digestion through a normal acid-base balance.

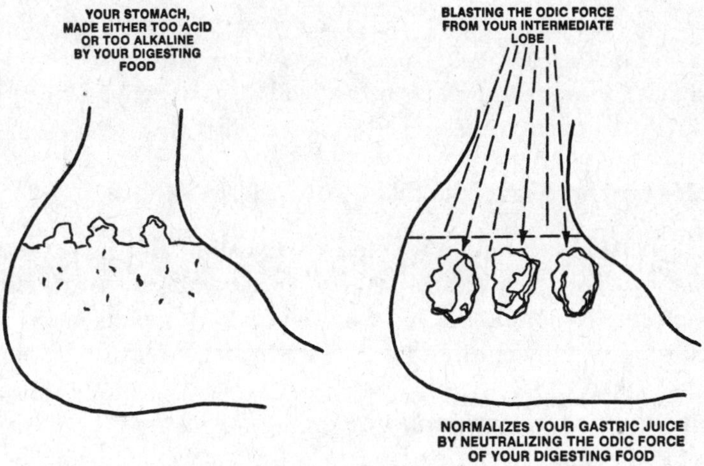

Illustration 7

How Your Unsuspected Habits Finish Off Your Liver

Your hidden liver ruiner is only half the story. You follow it up by finishing off your liver, even if you eat the best food, because you don't know what to do with your body after you eat. You very likely engage in vigorous activity or you move about quickly soon after eating. Or, you bend your body enough to contract your abdominal muscles and rush masses of blood from your alimentary tract to them. Or, you lie flat on your stomach and compress its contents. Or, you wear a belt, which strangles your abdomen as it makes room, during your meal, for the food and its digestion. Or, you eat snacks between meals and compel your digestion to continue unabated, flooding your stomach with hydrochloric acid. Or, you imbibe alcoholic drinks, soft drinks or fruit juices between meals. Your right side will distend with gas and distort your waistline, and your food will rush through you in a slightly diarrheal manner. You won't gain visible weight, just deadly fat which does not show up on the scale. Your congested liver will not secrete enough bile to digest your food fat, and the fat will infiltrate your liver and your other organs and form cholesterol plaques around the insides of your arteries.

One of the best ways to avoid this calamity is to be ultra-conscious of your body movements after you eat. (This is explored in depth in the last chapter). Also, eat raw garlic in your supper to increase your liver's bile secretion. Garlic also stimulates your peristalsis by the action of its etheric oils and helps your intestines to carry your partly digested food along your alimentary canal.

How Howard W. Was Soon Taken for a College Athlete

Howard W. fasted and dieted to stay slim. But he turned soft and flabby. He tried eating several meals a day instead, but his stomach turned sour and filled with gas and his bowels moved with difficulty. His face acquired lines of strain as his acidosis increased, and he looked older than his years.

By adopting the scientifically proved *Yogatronic Diet* and eating three square meals a day, Howard's bowels regained their regularity, and his waist shrank remarkably. With the added Triple Tonic Secret the lines of stress left his face. Before long, he looked so trim and youthful that he was repeatedly taken for a college athlete. "The *Yogatronic Diet,*" he exclaimed to me, "is the Fountain of Youth."

How Jesse B. Doubled his Company's Profits in Very Bad Times

Jesse B. was at his wits' end because times were so bad, inflation was so rampant and costs were so high that his company could not survive much longer. Besides, competition had grown keen. He was so discouraged that he lost interest in everything. His weight and waist, meanwhile, grew bigger and bigger.

The *Yogatronic Diet* allowed Jesse to fill himself—and yet reduce, while he felt stronger and younger. His insides slimmed and allowed his organs more room to function. He felt as if freed from a straight jacket, and new plans to save his company flashed into his mind. In a week, he found one that satisfied his associates, and they put it into operation. It did not seem to be magical at first, but the profits suddenly zoomed and saved the company. "The Triple Tonic Secret," he exclaimed, "adds a miracle power to the food I eat."

5

how yogatronics helps you to eliminate excess weight through the digestive tract—while eating all you want

Diet Secrets to Eat More, but get Thinner

For you to acquire a youthful trim body and a small waist, health has to remain your primary objective. You have to lose weight, but you lose weight *by adding more* of certain foods you eat, *not by cutting down* the amount you eat. When you eat too little, you not only feel weak but also bring on constipation. And constipation bulges your waist by increasing the amount of putrefied food it retains in your colon. Unless you take in a daily quantity of healthy bulk in your alimentary canal, you feel weak all over and your peristaltic wave lacks enough roughage to move your bowels easily and regularly.

Certain foods reduce you faster than others because they do not fatten you (they have a low caloric content) and because they keep your bowels regular. Others reduce you because they absorb your fat. The trouble is that you then reduce *all over*—even on your face and shoulders, so that your cheek-bones and collarbones show.

The foods that reduce your weight are not the foods that increase your weight. But they aren't lightweight foods, either. Foods that reduce you are the natural, healthy *bulky* foods. These fill your stomach, yet dump no fattening starch or sugar in your system. Their bulk passes through you, leaving no fatty accumulation behind. Healthy lightweight foods, such as grapes and honey, do not reduce you, because they contain sugar—even if it is in organic form. So they add to your body weight instead of reduce it. Leafy vegetables, celery and other components of a good food salad do not add weight to you, as they contain no sugar, although they do contain much healthy bulk. Carrots and beets, however, do contain some natural sugar. They should not be consumed in large quantities, but don't cut them out of your diet. Your health still remains your primary goal. Carrots are an excellent source of vitamin A (which you need for your skin and your eyes) and beets are an excellent blood builder that add color to your skin. Too many carrots every day, however, yellows your skin.

Other Cautions When Staying Slim

Avocados, coconuts and other oily fruits and nuts add weight, but don't cut them out altogether or your skin will turn dry and you will look old. Eat very little dried coconut, however, for it contains too much saturated fat and digests slowly. That is a pity, because it is an excellent nerve relaxer and endows you with physical power. Eat no more than a slice and a half of bread a day. To ensure bowel movement regularly, eat more prunes every day, but no more than five a day. Prunes contain oxalic acid and their extensive wrinkled surfaces retain too much sulfur preservative. The emptier your lower intestines are (as they will be when they move regularly), the more slender you look.

Why People Digest Differently

For dietary purposes, an enzyme is an organic substance secreted by your body cells which induces chemical changes in your foods but remains unchanged in the process. Vitamins do their work only in the presence of enzymes. Every vitamin is a part of an enzyme system. Enzymes are destroyed by cold and heat. That's why cooking or freezing your food is unwise. The temperature of your body, of course, never rises high enough to destroy your body's enzymes. As you grow older, however, the amount of hydrochloric acid in your stomach tends to diminish. You may then have trouble digesting proteins, because your supply of the protein-digesting enzyme pepsin cannot function in alkaline stomach.

The production of each enzyme also varies in effectiveness from person to person. One type of enzyme may be "strong" in you but "weak" in someone else. The intensity of all chemical reactions in your body varies from that in anybody else. Even those reactions taking place in any specific organ or tissue of your body will vary in efficiency between your body and someone else's. The very weights of the organs of different people called "normal" differ incredibly. Ranges of five to 10-fold are commonplace. The variation in the size of the esophagus might vary at least four-fold and importantly affect the ability of different people to swallow different foodstuffs. Thus, for you to eat fast or slow is a relative matter. Your eating speed even varies with your appetite for the particular meal.

How Your Normal Stomach Varies from Everybody Else's Normal Stomach

Your stomach, too, may vary markedly in size and shape from that of someone else. Some stomachs hold from 6 to 8 times more than others. That's why your eating habits and those of other people are not alike. It is normal for the stomach to be any of a large variety of shapes. Its very position in your body varies widely from that of many other "normal" people. (So does the position of your intestines and colon). The normal amount of pepsin (enzyme) you secrete in your stomach to digest protein may normally vary up to 449 times. In 5,000 individuals with healthy stomachs, the range varied up to an unbelievable *4300* times.

The older you get, as stated before, the less hydrochloric acid your stomach secretes. It may secrete as much as 23 percent less.

But your secretion and other people's don't diminish at the same rate. The amount secreted can vary still more if you are nervous and temperamental. Your very skin shows a difference in amounts of water-soluble vitamins. The difference may be two-fold for B_{12} and other vitamins, and more than five-fold for panthothenic acid. The variation in iron concentration, in contrast to other people, may range from two to 10 percent.

Digestion Differences Between You and Other Normal People

The zinc content of your blood is essential to the proper functioning of your pancreas, and it varies from 50 to 650 percent. A vitamin C deficiency may leave you susceptible to arsenicals and other poisons in your food. But, everybody is not equally susceptible to insecticides, even when they consume the same types of food from the same places for many years. Everybody in the afflicted areas, for instance, did not catch the black plague. The amount of vitamin C in the blood of normal people varies up to an amazing 155 times. Still other persons are healthy and suffer no symptoms when their tissues are saturated only with 50 percent of the average amount of the vitamin.

It is both impractical and impossible to test you for every digestion (or any other) difference between you and other normal people. But the fact that you differ from them, even when both of you are normal, compels you to adjust your differences to theirs, in order to get along with them. It is not easy to adjust your body in how to eat and exercise for you to maintain your best body weight and girth of waist. That's why you need the Triple Tonic Secret to help you.

A Significant Difference Between Your Stomach and Other Normal People's

An important effect, for instance, is the velocity with which your stomach passes its contents into your intestines. This velocity importantly controls your weight and the size of your waist. If your stomach does not digest your food sufficiently or satisfactorily, your intestinal digestion can make up for it, but your stomach will bulge noticeably for some time after your meals. You would have to remain inactive for a significantly longer period of time after your meals to permit this delayed digestion to take place, or you would risk developing serious stomach trouble. Your stomach would remain dilated and retain and ferment your food, and its movements and absorptive power would be reduced. You would eat more food but feel hungrier, and you would assimilate less of the food you eat. You would lose weight, even though you ate more and were less active, but you would acquire a larger waist. Even if you are normal, you can equalize these numerous differences of yours with the Triple Tonic Secret. Since the hydrochloric acid in your stomach varies more if you are nervous and temperamental, the Triple Tonic Secret is even more effective, in such cases, in controlling the efficiency of your digestion and dictating your weight and the size of your waist. So, practice this Triple Tonic Secret now. (Illus. 8).

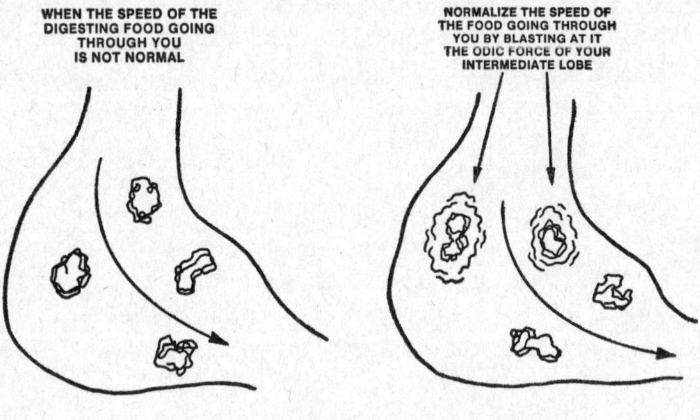

Illustration 8

Your Best Weight for a Youthful Look

You cannot eat foods that nourish you without adding calories to your body. Proteins and carbohydrates contain calories, and you can't exist without proteins and carbohydrates. Proteins also contain fats. Carbohydrates also turn to fat, unless they are used up in your body, which is most unlikely. It would require the mind of a god to figure out *exactly* how many extra calories you take in a day. You would have to record the *exact* amount of energy you expend all day long for the most insignificant moves, and you would end up a nervous wreck. Even dietetic foods have more calories (than necessary), reads the headline of a recent article in the *National Enquirer*.[1]

It is Impossible *Not* to Get Fat—Either Inside or Outside of You

No matter what you do, or how you eat, you are bound to get fat—even to get too much fat in your system. Fats furnish fat-soluble vitamins. Certain fatty acids are indispensable for your health and cannot be formed by your body. These, which were mentioned before, are linoleic, linolenic and arachidonic acids. Cholesterol (a fat) is needed by all your body cells and for producing hormones that regulate many of your body processes. Cholesterol is dangerous for you only when its intake is excessive, because it tends to form deposits in your arteries that can eventually set the stage for a heart attack. High sources of cholesterol are egg yolk, all dairy products such as milk (except skim milk), cheese and butter. Most meats, sweetbreads, liver and shellfish are also rich in cholesterol. Fish, poultry, nuts, beans and vegetables of all kinds are low in cholesterol. But meats are perfect proteins, while the other foods are not. The white meat of fowl, though, does not build up the muscles and power like lean "red" meat.

You also need unsaturated fat in your diet for your skin and for the sheaths that enclose and protect your nerves. You need it to fill the hollows of your face and neck, or you will look prematurely old. But keep your body weight "ideal," just as I keep mine. Keep it always within the range listed in the decades of researched and proved Table of "Ideal Weights" issued by the Metropolitan Life Insurance Company, on page 28.

The Secret is Wise Eating, not Dieting

For the average person, *Yogatronics* does not recommend diet. It recommends wise eating. Yet, teenage girls are dieting to death, announces Dr. Hilde Bruch, a psychiatrist at the Baylor College of Medicine in Houston, Texas. Some become as thin as "skeletons," their skin turns dry, their hair begins to fall out, their menstruation stops and they sleep very little. These girls claim that they are never tired, which is true, because their bodies burn up the protein in their muscles to make up for that which they should be getting from their food. So they feel light and limber, or "weightless." But they are throwing away their looks of youth and quickly turning into "old" women. They won't live longer, because they are also robbing protein from their heart muscles and growing weaker all over. The alteration of their figures will proceed so far and no more as these deluded girls continue dieting. But, their diet dooms them to looking older than they are if they keep it up, and it won't lengthen their lives for all the sacrifice.

To eat wisely and stay slim and healthy is to remain at your ideal weight every year all your life, like my wife and me. Eating wisely also hurls any further accumulating fat out of you before it can form the plaques inside your arteries or infiltrate the cells of your heart muscle. Following are the seven secrets to achieve these goals.

THE FIRST THREE SECRETS OF WISE EATING

Secret 1. Balance your diet, in order not to consume too many acid or alkaline foods at any one meal. You don't need to compute the calories or follow a special menu. Just eat meat or fowl (protein) at the same meal at which you eat salads, or vice versa. Do so twice a day, anyway.

Secret 2. Let one meal a day (say, lunch) consist wholly of fruits, a staying starchy food (like potatoes) and some dates if you expect to work hard or be very active after lunch. Fruits will control your weight, but they also add fiber to your diet and reduce the acidity of your stomach. However, they provide you with a fast-absorbed sugar which fills you promptly with energy but which also leaves you quickly, and you will feel weak less than two hours later. Bananas and potatoes, in contrast, provide you with a slowly absorbed sugar which stays with you for hours and keeps you feeling strong for the rest of the day. Yet, they still hold down your weight. Bananas even satisfy your craving for sweets.

Secret 3. For supper, eat another balanced diet consisting of a complete protein (like meat), with an alkaline salad to balance it and prevent your stomach from turning acid. An acid stomach, as you already know, contributes to a bad skin, constipation and a bulging waist. It causes undesirable weight gain because its natural contraction and relaxation and the resulting peristaltic wave are retarded. You turn lazy and lethargic, skip your daily exercise (or do less of it) and grow flabby and fatter.

THE SECOND THREE SECRETS OF WISE EATING

Secret 4. The fiber in your diet tends to sweep out the fat in your food before it is absorbed by your body and eliminates it through your bowels. Drinking water between meals (about 8 glasses a day) helps additionally because the fiber absorbs water.

Don't, however, overconsume fibrous food. It can give you maddening gripes, as well as absorb too many trace minerals from your food. In this respect, however, it also absorbs arsenic, mercury and other insecticides on your food after your saliva and your gastric juice saturate it.

Secret 5. If you have the opportunity where you live or work to vigorously climb several flights of stairs a day, do so. But don't do it for two and a half hours after breakfast or one and a half hours after a "light" lunch. Climbing stairs, especially by twos, will absorb the fat from your body much faster than jogging, tennis, handball or any other activity. As stated before, it uses up several times the amount of energy which those other activities do, in far less time.

Secret 6. Again, have no snacks between meals, not even fruit juices. They turn your stomach acid and delay the onward movement of your digesting food, which is propelled by its bulk. As a consequence, your alimentary tract absorbs more of the fat in your food. A daily routine of three square meals a day promotes a diurnal tide in your alimentary canal which conditions the muscles of your stomach and intestines to contract stronger during your digestion than they normally would. The fiber in your food, as a consequence, sweeps more fat out of your digestive tract daily, even if you eat the same amount of it, and controls your weight more effectively.

THE LAST SECRET OF WISE EATING

Secret 7. Don't be misled by assertions that several small meals a day reduces you faster than three square meals. They won't, because your stomach will have to digest food for hours on end and be acid all that time. The onward movement of your digesting food will be slower, because your stomach and intestines will get little rest between meals. They lose the dynamic power of triggering peristaltic waves regularly. Besides, if your meals are not big enough, they won't distend your stomach and intestines sufficiently to let your food be pushed on faster. More than three meals a day produces an unusual amount of gas in your alimentary tract, forces you to be unusually active too soon after meals and overburdens your heart by compelling it, during most of the day, to supply blood to your digestive organs and your muscles at the same time. Your heart works 48 percent harder when you are digesting. When you add the effort of muscular activity or exercise to it, you overburden it. Besides, your alimentary tract will be supplied with less blood to digest and absorb your food because so much of it will be diverted to your muscles. Much of your food will pass through you undigested and unabsorbed, and it will putrefy and fill you with pockets of gas which will distend your waist.

I disagree with those who oppose three square meals a day on the fallacious promise that nibbling the same amount of food in small quantities throughout the day will cause you to lose weight. Wild animals in their natural habitats do eat without regularity and maintain their normal weights, but they have to hunt and catch their food. The caged animal does not. Your stomach and intestines, furthermore, don't stretch permanently to make room for "large meals" three times a day, because those organs do not stretch permanently. Of course, don't overeat fatty foods at any meal. Instead, consume enough fibrous food at each square meal to fill you, before you stuff yourself with fat.

Never Use Cooking Oil

Actually, the cause of much overweight in America is the habit of habitual snacking, of eating six times a day, as so many people do. Some snackers nibble up to 20 times a day. According to Food and Nutrition News, this is not unusual among adults, especially among women between 25 and 45. Such a routine is encouraged by the wide variety of snack foods available at sporting events, in stores, restaurants and vending machines. The article adds that the growing trend in the United States is toward more skipping of meals, eating less meals at the table, of gobbling more convenience foods—and more snacking. Steer clear of such habits and follow my three-meals-a-day routine with balanced acid-alkaline meals containing fiber. You will then, as so many of my disciples and myself are doing, retain your "ideal" weight indefinitely. You will be in the best digestive health and continuously at your physical and mental peak.

How Charles F. and his Wife "Ate Like Horses," but Still Wore Youthful Clothes in their Sixties

For years, Charles F. and his wife combatted their weight problems. They tried one diet after another, cut out certain foods altogether from their diets and engaged in different sports. All of these methods worked—to a degree—but required considerable self-denial, thinned down their faces too much and also reduced the regions of their bodies which they wanted to keep full.

With the wide-ranging *Yogatronic Diet* Charles and his wife found that they could fill themselves at meal times, and yet thin down in the right places but not so much in the others. Although they were in their sixties, they were wearing youthful clothes again in a few weeks and looking younger than they had for twenty years. Regularly when they ate, of course, they projected the Triple Tonic Secret within them into their food.

How Thelma Z. Lost Her Matronly Look Speedily

Thelma Z. despaired of ever getting a second husband. She was divorced and had two teen-aged children who were soon going to college, and she envisioned a lonely "aging life" ahead for herself. She had filled out too much all over. Although she was not "big and fat," as she termed it, she had lost what she considered "the appeal of the young things" to excite men romantically.

With the *Yogatronic Diet* and the Triple Tonic Secret Thelma "wasped" her figure in four short weeks and changed her whole romantic outlook. A few months later she remarried.

REFERENCES

[1]*National Enquirer*. Nov. 15, 1977.

6

how to slenderize with yogatronics through heart-strengthening foods

What I Knew 55 Years Before Science Proved It

"Seven million of us have heart disease." That is the estimate from the Center for Health Statistics. "No longer can heart disease be considered a problem of age." That is the warning of Dr. Edward Kass of the Harvard Medical School.

I knew that from the age of 10, 55 years before science when, against the advice of so many people, I competed in track and spent my Saturdays climbing up and down the steep Ancon Hill in the Canal Zone. I boxed regularly and did "road work" (jogging long distances) for boxing endurance all through seventh and eighth grades, high school and half of dental school. I lifted weights for six years, before stopping to do my own non-apparatus exercises. At the age of 35, I competed in Illinois in the 100-yard dash in national meets, against world record holders from twelve to fifteen years my juniors. I also competed in state amateur swimming meets against state champions aged 16 to 21. In body building at the age of 40, (as described in Chapter 1), with only six weeks brief training without weights or apparatus, I competed in a state championship meet against a field of body builders half my age and was selected as a finalist along with the youth who became the holder of all the amateur world physique titles. And remember, I did not join the physique champions in taking high-protein pills to get bigger and trimmer. I confined myself only to grocery and supermarket food. I have continued exercising regularly and have written a number of courses and books about physical fitness.

The Proof of the Pudding Is: I Look About Half of, and Feel About One-Fourth of, My Age

From the age of 10, in other words, I already logically and psychically disagreed with the longevity rules of the top scientists of the day. I have never changed my mind, but have continued exercising ever since, just as vigorously as ever. I will never stop doing so. I feel as spry today as I did at 10. In the meantime, I have observed person after person whom I knew well or read about, who either warned me in person or in print against the "dangers" of exercise and its developing an "athletic heart," die off like flies. I, however, live on and on, hardly looking any older than I did thirty years ago (according to those who knew me then), and exercising as strenously today as I did at twenty-one.

My heart and lungs, after all that, are as strong as Hercules'. I never suffered from heart disease, proving that the present discovery by science that your heart gets stronger from exercise is absolutely true. Fortunately for me, I was convinced of that from the age of 10—convinced that I could compete against anybody of any age, no matter how long I lived. I do not tell you this to prove I was a 10-year-old Einstein, but to show you that having hit upon these truths so remarkably early, my whole life-style of nutrition and health care has already been subjected to a lifetime of testing.

Diet Secrets to Shrink Your Waist and Revitalize Your Heart

After all these decades, the consensus of specialists in the field is that there are *six important ways* to help prevent early heart attack. These are: (1) Stop smoking. (2) Keep blood pressure low. (3) Maintain lean body weight. (4) Eat a low-fat diet. (5) Exercise prudently. (6) Take time to relax.

Five of these six rules are *the exact ones* which I have taught my readers and students to follow for a long and healthy life. I disagree heartily with the sixth rule, and proved how right I was in the last chapter of my last book, ZODIC FORCE CONTROL: SECRET OF MIRACLE HEALING AND LONG LIFE. That chapter contains a thorough description of the longest and most elucidating revolutionary health experiment of all time, which I have inadvertently conducted with a long-time friend from our early twenties to the present.

THE FIRST FIVE RULES

Rule 1. Stop Smoking. Smoking between meals, or in fact at any time, is no better for you than snacking. Your lungs take in air to purify your blood. If, instead, you inhale nicotinized smoke, your blood does not purify but becomes increasingly acid. Acidic blood carries large amounts of body waste and puts a severe strain on your heart. So you smoke more, to stimulate yourself. Even if you only exhale the smoke, the air around you reeks with it, and you inhale it anyway. Non-smokers near you fare no better. They, too, have to inhale your smoke if they are to breathe at all. Twenty years after I first proposed this theory, science finally announced the veracity of this assertion, which classifies it as another important miracle discovery.

Rule 2. Keep your blood pressure low. When your system is overacid, it is unhealthy. It is full of poison and exhausts itself trying to cast off the poison. Overacidity probably erodes your vital organs, including your heart, and your blood vessels, just as acid fruits erode your teeth. This erosion takes place slowly, as with the teeth, but eventually its effects appear. An overacid diet is invariably present in such conditions as acid stomach, constipation, ulcers, cirrhosis of the liver, gallstones, kidney stones, hemorrhoids, arthritis, rheumatism, sinus trouble and kindred common complaints. Your nerves are irritated by your acid blood, and you become jumpy and overexcitable, which keeps your blood pressure high. In the end, you come down with a degenerative disease, such as heart disease. As you already know, most fruits and vegetables are alkaline food which can be used to keep your blood pressure low and protect you against heart disease.

I condemn the use of seasoning (which includes salt) for any food, as well as sugar. The Louisiana State University School of

Medicine has shown that a combination of sugar and salt in a meal developed high blood pressure in monkeys. High blood pressure is even being reported in school children who eat the junk-food combination of soft drink, potato chips and hamburger, which so many of them favor. Wise eating and the amount of fruit recommended by the *Yogatronic Diet* will keep your blood pressure low and reduce the risk of heart attack.

Rule 3. Maintain lean body weight. Today I weigh *exactly* what I did at 20, in my physical prime, when I engaged in my last boxing bout, and I am still all muscle. I refuse to confess my actual age, because I think of myself always as 28.

Rule 4. Eat a low-fat diet. The *Yogatronic Diet* outlines the general features of the alkaline diet to train you to use it to balance your meals properly. Thus, you can enjoy your meals and be healthy—and help yourself *retain* your youthful look.

Again, most fresh fruits and vegetables are alkaline foods. Such foods contain practically no fat, or the least fat of all foods. Acid foods satisfy your appetite faster because they stimulate the taste glands to secrete faster. Sugar becomes acid through chemical reaction and turns your stomach acid. Over-acidity also brings torpidity of brain and muscle. It poisons your blood (which raises your blood pressure) and tissues (since your blood runs through your tissues) and leaves you lazy and easily fatigued, all of which limits your activity and fattens your waist. Alkalizing yourself with lemon juice in the morning clears your brain, because the vagus nerve which runs from your brain to your stomach carries the effects of your stomach conditions to your brain. This alkalinity also gets into your muscles, including your heart muscle, and restores their health and vigor by neutralizing their acidity.

Rule 5. Exercise prudently. You know that I have been exercising systematically since the age of 10. But, I have striven not to break records and possibly injure my heart. I elaborated about this in several of my past books, from 2 to 23 years before science.

I was already teaching these five rules to prevent heart disease in *Solar Diet*, 23 years before science discovered them and gave them official approval in one package. That's why my readers and students are kept far ahead of their time.

Rule 6. DO NOT take time to relax. Science has not yet found this last miracle discovery of mine. It still believes that meditation and relaxation prolong the life of your heart or prevent heart disease, just as it believed for most of the last fifty-five years that exercise shortened life, that you lived long by exercising very little, if at all, and only strained your heart if you did. I was correct in disbelieving that, and I insist that I am also correct in disagreeing with *their* Rule 6 now. I have my own physique and health and heart to prove it. In the 43-year real life experiment, which I describe in *Zodic Force Control*, I prove that your heart is strongest when you throw your mind into the rapture of *zodic ecstasy*, not into meditation and relaxation.

THE MAGIC REABSORPTION POWER OF PLANT FIBER

The heart disease rate for vegetarians is 6 times lower than in the general population.[1] It was proven that:

1. People who eat plant fiber in the form of vegetables, fruits and cereals with bran and whole wheat bread, suffer less from heart disease.
2. Plant fiber is more effective in lowering blood cholesterol than substituting polyunsaturates for animal fat.
3. When the fiber moves through your small and lower intestines it carries out the bile your liver produced and the cholesterol your food contained.

The fiber, in other words, prevents your digestion from reabsorbing these "potentially dangerous" compounds. Dr. William Sherman, biochemist and director of nutrition research for the National Live Stock and Meat Board, consequently advises you to eat fresh fruits and vegetables every day and to substitute fresh fruits for processed fruits. He urges you to eat the whole orange rather than drink the juice. He also encourages you to include a salad and vegetable for lunch and dinner.[2]

How Liquor Affects Your Heart, According to Revolutionary Scientific Research

Yogatronics recommends *no liquor.* Liquor of any kind is a stomach acidifier. Beer and wine not only turn it acid, but put on fat-weight. Fat fills up the insides of your arteries, contributing to the possibilities of your falling victim to an early stroke. Wine is hailed by some as a great blood builder, but its alcohol content is a fast stomach acidifier. Fresh beets, raisins, liver and beefsteak can build up your blood fast enough. Since it heats the body fast, in an emergency, wine can revive you, or even ward off the sudden onset of a cold, but don't take it as a regular part of your diet. Harsher liquors, like whiskey, should be avoided completely. A hangover is actually a serious acid stomach.

Twenty-three years later, in the September, 1977 issue of the *New England Journal of Medicine*, a study was published involving 7,075 men living in Honolulu, by Dr. Abraham Kagan and Dr. George Rhoads, covering a six-year span. The doctors discovered that drinking three or more beers a day, or two shots of liquor, *can reduce your prospects of having a heart attack by more than fifty percent*. It was an astounding discovery, they concluded. It had been commonly accepted, they stated, that heavy drinkers, for one reason or another, don't suffer from heart disease. But it had never been suspected that such was also the case with people on low intakes of liquor. The obvious conclusion, they went on, was that the people who drank were less likely to suffer heart attacks than those who did not drink. The researchers believed that there might be some connection between alcohol in the system and the body's synthesis of alpha cholesterol. (According to recent discoveries, alpha cholesterol is a *beneficial* form of cholesterol). They also believed that alcohol simultaneously lowered beta cholesterol, the kind of cholesterol in the body which is connected with heart disease.

Liquor and Heart Stress

Fortunately, the researchers warned the public that they could *not* advise anyone to drink without caution, particularly more than three beers a day. They were dealing with new ground, they emphasized, or with very new discoveries. They did not remind the public, however, of the research, published a month earlier, that exercise cuts male heart patients' death rate in half. The Vancouver cardiologist, Dr. Arthur Dodek, citing a supervised exercise program from NASA studies, added that the program brought on a lower resting heart rate, lower blood pressure, increased stamina, a feeling of better health, reduced the weight and reduced stress and tension.[3] I had revealed these effects on stress and tension to a close friend in a personal letter forty years before.

Note: As this book goes to press, Dr. Ernest P. Noble, director of the National Institute on Alcohol Abuse and Alcoholism, announced that "even moderate amounts of alcohol consumption can subject your heart to stress and cause heart disease. He even disagrees with the contention that alcohol is a good tranquilizer. You would have to drink enough to be drunk, he explained, which he could not recommend as a beneficial sedative. Under the influence of alcohol, he went on, some people only become aggressive or fall into a state of depression.

How Revolutionary Scientific Research Overlooked the Blatant Facts

The researchers had overlooked two most important features in interpreting their discovery. They had not pointed out that alcohol considerably reduced the appetite so that the drinker happened to eat less cholesterol-forming food or that since the typical non-drinker ate *more food* than the alcoholic (and much of it was "junk" food), he happened to eat more cholesterol-forming foods than the drinker. No wonder he suffered a greater chance of heart attack than the alcoholic!

Even monkeys, as a recent study by the Louisiana State University School of Medicine showed, developed a high blood pressure when fed what children ate. The typical child, the researchers found, ingested 34 percent of his calories as snacks, which were high in salt and sugar. Not being a drinker, he ate more "junk" food.

The researchers also did not mention the finding in the previous year that the heart attack rate for vegetarians was *six times* lower than in other people, which included those who drank beer, wine, or *any kind of liquor*. Like so many scientific conclusions, theirs was not based on all the facts at hand. Their announcement probably boosted the liquor industry, but it did not help drinkers who took it at its face value.

Alcohol and Long Life

So, I repeat with more determination than ever that *Yogatronics* recommends *no liquor*. I also submit that the irritation of liquor on the stomach can cause gastritis, ulcers, liver dysfunction, deficiency of vitamin B_1, damage to the nervous system, rapid heart beat, eye pathologies, decreased mental acuity and other catastrophic physiological effects. Liquor also *fattens* the body, even when your scales hardly change. As I wrote earlier in this book, alcohol increases your appetite at first, by stimulating more secretion of hydrocholoric acid by your stomach. (But that also increases your stomach acidity). On the other hand, it *lowers* the formation of the protein-digesting enzyme, pepsin, in your stomach, thereby lessening the amount of protein your stomach digests. The amount of undigested protein moving along your digestive tract is increased as a result. It is putrefied and excreted and leaves your body protein-starved. Therefore, your heart muscle is also starved. That's why alcohol actually does *not* lengthen the life of your heart. Besides, all regular beer-drinkers put on fatty weight and acquire a typical "beer belly," which hardly leaves them "youthful and trim." Their livers also get fat.

How to Cut Your Risk of Heart Disease in Half

An investigation conducted in three separate studies by top researchers claims that calcium supplements taken four times a day reduce cholesterol levels faster than exercise, drugs or improved diets. They insist, furthermore, that there are no side effects, as there would be with drugs.[4] They announce that the calcium can dramatically reduce fat and cholesterol levels in your blood and diminish your risk of heart disease by as much as 50 percent.

Such a procedure might be suitable for the hospitalized patient, but I would not recommend it to any reader or student of mine with normal health. For one thing, taking as concentrated a product as calcium supplements into your system four times a day abuses the soft linings of your stomach and can lead to stomach trouble, or even ulcers. Being a stony material, it may curse you with granite-bowels, constipating you and causing hemorrhoids. Such a way of eating won't bring you a flat, small waist either, although the researchers might not consider that fact significant.

The Natural Way to Lengthen the Life of Your Heart

The researchers do admit that you can get your daily requirement of calcium by eating at least one serving each of skim milk, low-fat cheese and a fresh vegetable. But they urge you to *double* your daily calcium intake by adding another 800 mg. with calcium carbonate pills. Well, the *Yogatronic Diet* already doubles the daily calcium intake by specifying a daily intake of *two* servings of skim milk instead of one, and *two* servings of salad consisting of fresh vegetables instead of one. The *Yogatronic Diet* also approves of cheese for *gaining* weight, and such cheese contains three and a half times the calcium of nonfat (cottage) cheese. The high fiber content of the two servings of salads it advises daily reduces considerably the amount of fat in the cheese.

When I was close to fifty, I had an X-ray taken of my right hand to examine an old boxing injury. The head physician of the clinic remarked in astonishment that my bones contained as much calcium as a *youth's*. My natural method of getting daily calcium had passed the undisputed clinic test gloriously. So, those daily foods had certainly supplied *twice* the amount of the daily calcium intake recommended by the researchers "just to be safe." They caused me no side effects and did not require me to take calcium carbonate, which may form "fecal stones."

By cutting your risk of heart attack in half, you can remain more active than otherwise, can exercise more, and can more easily acquire and retain a trim youthful body and a small waist.

How the Yogatronic Diet Protects You More from Heart Disease.

It was found in experiments with rats that your sympathetic nervous system stimulates you less intensely when you fast. It regains its diminished intensity and raises your body heat beyond normal when you feed yourself again and add sucrose (sugar) to your diet. According to the researchers (Young and Landsbury), the signal which your body gives your sympathetics to regain their lost intensity is unknown. But, they conclude, a connection seems to exist between the raising of your body heat wtih your diet and the resulting increased stimulation of your sympathetics and heart disease.

That's obviously why an alkaline diet holds down the risks of a vegetarian suffering a heart attack to one-sixth that of a non-vegetarian. An alkaline diet produces comparatively little body heat; it therefore does not intensify the activitiy of your sympathetic nervous system. (Intensifying it would raise your blood pressure). That's another unexpected benefit derived from following the predominantly alkaline *Yogatronic Diet*. The Triple Tonic Secret supplies the unknown signal to your sympathetics to keep down their intensities closer to those they assume when you fast, and thus keep your heart healthier.

The Necessary Calcium-Phosphorus Ratio for Strong Heart and Health

Phosphorus is abundant in your foods, and you have little likelihood of suffering from a deficiency of it. The opposite is true of calcium. Yet, its ratio to phosphorus in your food intake has an important influence on the metabolism of both calcium and phosphorus within your body. If your food lacks enough of one, your body will not utilize the other one properly, even if the normal amount of it is present in your food. If you are an adult, your calcium intake should be close to equal that of your phosphorus. (In a growing child it should be twice that of phosphorus). If you eat lots of cereals, nuts and legumes (beans, peas, and other vegetables of that class) you ingest considerable phosphorus in a chemical combination known as phytic acid. Phytic acid combines with the calcium in your food and removes it from your body. But phosphorus cannot be called a villain, because you need it to use fat properly, to combine with your protein so that it digests, and to help digest important B vitamins. Phosphorus is also a significant substance in your brain tissue.

To absorb the phosphorus, however, your body needs quite a bit of calcium *at the same time*. You need vitamin D (or a regular amount of sunshine) in order to absorb either the calcium or the phosphorus. Your body does not use the phosphorus in your food otherwise. But, since most foods contain more phosphorus than calcium, it is difficult to find enough foods which have more calcium than phosphorus. That's why bone meal is sometimes offered as a solution. I am not criticising bone meal, but I prefer plain food. Man has never lived off bones, so I am not sure that his digestive system can handle such an intake on a regular basis. That's why I have searched extensively for foods which contain substantial proportions of calcium over phosphorus and have drawn up a table. (Table 1.) Some foods listed, like baking powders, candied citron,

Table 1

Foods That Have a Considerable Margin of Calcium over Phosphorus

Baking powders
Beet greens, raw
Cabbage (pakchoi)
Carob flour (St. John's bread)
Chard, Swiss
Cheese, natural
Citron, candied
Collards
Cream substitute (skim milk, lactose)
Dandelion greens
Fennel, Common
Horseradish, raw
Kale
Kumquats
Lemon peel, raw
Lettuce (leaf and romaine)
Loganberries
Molasses
Mustard greens
Mustard spinach
Okra
Olives
Oranges (with peel*—more calcium)
Pudding mix
Rennin tablets
Salad dressing (Italian regular)
Sauerkraut
Sauerkraut juice, canned
Seaweeds (Agar, Irish moss, & kelp)
Sesame seeds, whole
Syrups
Sugar, brown & maple
Turnip greens
Vinespinach, raw
Watercress

**Note*: Keep away from orange peel. The yellow outside portion turns your skin yellow, as from jaundice. It is also concentrated with poisonous sprays. In addition, both the yellow outside and the white inside of the skin contain so much fiber that they can bring on a severe attack of gripes because your alimentary tract won't digest them.

orange peel, pudding mix, rennin tablets, and sugar, I definitely do not recommend. I listed them only because they, too, contain far more calcium than phosphorus. I advise you to include some of these foods regularly in your meals to avoid taking in too little calcium daily, affecting your heart and weakening your muscles. When your muscles weaken, your activity lessens, you exercise less and you gain weight and enlarge your waist. Your life is thereby shortened. Keep the ratio of your calcium-phosphorus daily intake as close to the proper level as possible.

How to Enjoy Fat-Heavy Foods and Hardly Fear Heart-Attack or Stroke

Scientists have recently announced that "eating onions may reduce heart attack risks." Dr. A. S. Truswell, professor of the Queen Elizabeth College of London University, the conductor of the research, called the discovery "amazing." Dr. Frederic Stare, a physician and professor of the Harvard School of Public Health, declared, after studying the findings, that when eaten with a high-fat meal, onions possibly reduce the risk of stroke or heart attack, which is a constant threat after the consumption of such a meal.

Dr. Stare added that other similar work confirmed to a degree that the eating of onions with a fatty meal tended to influence the clotting power of the blood. The fatty meal facilitated the forming of a blood clot and contributed to the possibility of a stroke or heart attack. If subsequent studies, he concluded, demonstrate that onions tend to reduce the clotting power of the blood, they would be evidence that onions do help to decrease the chances of suffering a heart attack.

Over twenty-four years ago, I had already taught my readers to add onions and garlic to the heavy dish of their meal. I described meat as being the important requirement for a heavy food, and meat (except lean meat) is a fat-heavy food. Onions and garlic, I pointed out, helped to purify the blood. Since purifying the blood obviously amounts to reducing its ability to form blood clots, I was giving my readers a life-prolonging, or even a life-saving, piece of advice *that far back*, without being aware of it. Over a period of 24 years it may have prolonged or even saved the lives of many of them.

The Triple Tonic Secret for Strengthening Your Heart when You Eat

In perfectly normal young men their heartbeats ranged from 43 to 103 beats per minute. Normal hearts varied, in pumping capacity, from 3.16 to 10.81.[5] In order to strengthen your heart the most from your food, strive to increase your *absorption* of healthy heart food. Your absorption of it varies widely with how you think when you eat. Several times, while you eat, follow Illustration 9.

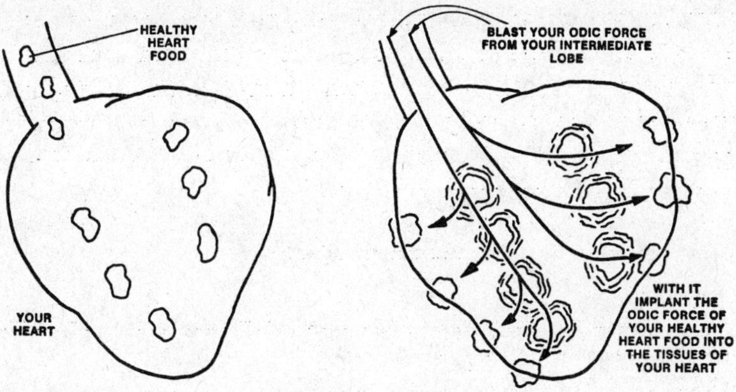

Illustration 9

How Kevin L. Altered His Weight and Pioneered a Wealth-Making Enterprise

Kevin L. fatigued easily under pressure. He was about 50 pounds overweight and it added an extra burden on his heart. I explained to him that a big waist lessened the space for his heart and lungs to function normally. His diaphragm, also, could not expand as much as it should, and fat accumulated around and within his heart. His arteries narrowed with cholesterol deposits and forced his heart to strain to drive his blood through them. He had exciting plans ahead for his business but doubted if he had the energy to carry them through.

With the *Yogatronic Diet* Kevin shed his excess weight in a natural manner, faster than he ever had. Since he did not have to curb his appetite, he still felt full after each meal. But, he also felt strong because his waist shrank and his heart and lungs regained their normal functioning room. His enthusiasm for his business zoomed. Four years later, it was grossing almost a million dollars a year.

How Enid T. Lost 30 Lbs. and Became Irresistible

Enid T. yearned for a glamor career, but she couldn't stay slim enough. Different diets removed much of her weight, but they weakened her and sapped her efforts to be glamorous. If she could only, she pleaded with me, feel as lively as when she weighed 10 pounds more!

The *Yogatronic Diet* solved Enid's problem. She lost weight even faster than before, in a natural way, but felt stronger and retained her sparkle. The Triple Tonic Secret seemed to strengthen her heart, and she even started to exercise. She made a stunning success with her glamor career, and the vice-president of her company proposed to her.

REFERENCES

[1]Researchers of the Loma Linda University School of Health in California, October, 1974. *National Enquirer;* Oct. 26, 1976.

[2]*National Enquirer*, Aug. 7, 1974.

[3]The Vancouver cardiologist, Dr. Arthur Dokek, citing a study of the Cardiopulmonary Research Institute in Seattle, *National Enquirer*, July 6, 1977.

[4]Dr. Marvin Bierenbaum, director of the Atherosclerosis Research Group at St. Vincent's Hospital in Montclair, N.J. *National Enquirer*, Feb. 1, 1977.

[5]*Biochemical Individuality: The Basis for the Genetotrophic Concept.* R. J. Williams, The University of Texas at Austin. Austin and London, Fifth printing, 1975.

7

Cholesterol Magic with Yogatronics

Alpha-Cholesterol, the Wonderful Beneficial Cholesterol

In the last chapter it was stated that researchers believe that alcohol cuts the chances of a heart attack by altering the physiology of the drinker to produce alpha-cholesterol, the beneficial form of cholesterol. Very early in 1977, top medical researchers made the startling discovery that *alpha*-cholesterol affected the heart in just the *opposite* manner of beta-cholesterol, the enemy of the heart, and had a *reverse effect* on heart disease.[1] Alpha-cholesterol seemed to cart beta-cholesterol through the blood into the liver, where it was eliminated.

The big question then arose: How could you build up your level of blood alpha-cholesterol? Dr. Castelli (the researcher) replied that it could be done through running and other exercises, indicating that long distance runners had an ample supply of it.

Another leading researcher, Dr. Wissler,[2] added that you could raise your alpha-cholesterol in several ways: (1) With a diet low in saturated fats; that is, by eating less meat, eggs and butterfat. (2) Also, by eating more fresh fruits, vegetables, fish and fowl. The vegetables should be eaten raw or steamed. (3) He specifically recommended green vegetables like peas, spinach and lettuce. He especially favored carrots and celery because of their high fiber content. (4) He went on to recommend nearly any fresh fruit, including apples, oranges and peaches. (5) He warned against bananas because of their "high fat content." (6) And, he recommended avoidance of canned fruits packed with syrup. (7) Any kind of fish, he said, was good, like trout or perch. (8) He cautioned against shellfish like shrimp, lobster or crab. (9) He called turkey and chicken the best fowl to consume, but limited it to the white meat because it had less fat than the dark meat.

Dr. George Rhoads, associate professor of public health at the University of Hawaii, agreed that the more alpha-cholesterol you had, the less your chances were of having heart disease.

The Magic Discoveries in Yogatronics

For the *Yogatronic Diet*, I list the eating of foods which *do* produce alpha-cholesterol and describe what they do to your body. But *Yogatronics* goes even further and lists foods which the scientists caution *against* for alpha-cholesterol. I explain how these foods are necessary if you wish to build up into an attractive person physically with shape, and yet be trim. I also reveal, however, what foods to add to such wise eating to counteract any deleterious effects. Here are the explanations of the ways to build alpha-cholesterol together with the diet wisdom I have accumulated over the years. It is climaxed with the Triple Tonic Secret to further increase your alpha-cholesterol. Let us compare the *Yogatronic Diet* with Dr. Wissler's nine ways to build alpha-cholesterols in the blood.

First Way. A Diet Low in Saturated Fats

Start your supper with a lighter plate, like a salad. Above all, don't wreck your salad with any of the salad dressings composed of condiments, vinegar and oil. Raw onion, sliced very thin, also adds taste to the salad. To the heavy dish (protein) add garlic and onions whenever possible. Garlic is the natural, germ-killing and blood-purifying food.

The medical use of garlic dates back at least to 1550 B.C. The Egyptians used it for twenty-two ailments, including headaches and heart problems. Recently, a team of physicians from the University of Benghazi, Libya[3] found that garlic lowered the blood cholesterol of animals with arteriosclerosis by as much as 51 percent. It appreciably reduced the hardening of their arteries and helped prevent the formation of cholesterol plaques in the inner walls of their arteries. While science laughed at garlic back in 1933, I already believed in it and ate it daily. In the 1940s, its power was established when Dr. Arthur Stoll, a Nobel Prize winner, found that the herb contained the bacteria-killing mineral allium. By writing in *Solar Diet* that garlic was a "blood purifying food" I obviously meant that garlic reduced whatever was in the blood that harmed the body. We now know that that would include cholesterol, toxins, fats and other biochemical compounds and wastes which injure the health and the heart.

First Way (Continued). Eat Less Meat and Eggs

I did not, and still don't, agree much with that warning. Meat is the favorite heavier supper food. Vegetarians do not believe in meat, but meat is a fine food. I once lived for six years as a vegetarian. It supercharged me with energy like a mystic and helped to cure me of many ailments. But it thinned me down by forty pounds. It obviously filled me with alpha-cholesterol and absolutely favored my heart. A diet with meat helped restore my lost weight, although it brought back many of my chronic ailments. It obviously reduced some of my alpha-cholesterol. I overcame these conditions again by introducing fresh garlic, and natural vitamin-mineral food supplements to my diet, which I ceased taking eighteen years ago, although I have remained just as healthy, and still kept my weight. So, I obviously regained my full alpha-cholesterol, but this time I retained my natural weight and normal appearance.

To limit yourself to a vegetarian diet, then, is unnecessary, providing you regularly eat vegetables (without devitalizing them further) with your meat and (possibly) food supplements. But, I repeat, I stopped the food supplements eighteen years ago, after taking them for six years. You don't have to thin yourself down to a skeleton to be in good health. Eat meat for supper and enjoy it. Get the protein it brings you. Meat, after all, is *the* complete protein. It contains *all* the essential amino acids. Meat, too, will help burn up the excess body fat of the overweight individual. Of course, the meat must be lean.

Note: I heartily recommend eggs—one a day (not fried). I have eaten eggs every day for 90 precent of my life and am in perfect health. I am convinced that the lecithin in eggs does a tremendous job of nullifying any deleterious effects of the cholesterol in the egg yolk. My wife, my private disciple and others are doing very well, too. I urge no one, of course, to eat them against his professional healer's recommendation. In fact, the three of us alternate with 1 egg one day, and 2 eggs the next day, all year round.

The Warming, Energizing Finisher

Your breakfast is not complete without the warming, energizing finisher. Milk, warmed to a degree, is better than coffee, tea or chocolate. If overweight is your problem, don't eliminate milk from your diet. Skim milk contains everything in whole milk except the fattening butterfat. Both liquid and powdered milk solids are available in most food stores. Drying the milk must deplete it somewhat of vitamins, which are destroyed by heat or light. So, fresh skim milk, of course, is the better of the two. The important thing is to *keep milk in your diet*. Professor Thomas Richardson of the University of Wisconsin, a food scientist, announces that, according to recent research, milk contains factors that somehow prevent cholesterol from building up in the blood. Drinking milk, he states, has reduced cholesterol levels. Milk is a valuable food and cannot be left out of your diet.

Without knowing that milk reduced blood cholesterol, I refused to believe the warnings against it by science for the last three decades and have continued to drink it daily and to recommend it highly. There is also a psychic element behind my miracle discoveries which guides me to the right decision, even when it is absolutely against the findings of the most advanced thinkers of the time.

Second Way to Raise Your Alpha-Cholesterol. Eat More Fresh Fruits and Vegetables, Fish and Fowl

I recommend that two of your meals a day contain fresh fruits and vegetables. Chicken, duck and other game birds are good food, too, although they don't build up your blood or your muscles like animal meat. But, unless too fat, they are easy to digest. They don't turn your stomach acid, bloat you with gas or pass through you partly undigested. The fatter the meat the harder it is for your stomach to digest it. The kind of meat you eat, also, is important. The so-called "red" meats: lean beef, veal, mutton and lamb are very good. Liver, kidneys, brains and tripe are the very best meats for you, but cattle for market are now fed antibiotics and a host of other chemicals. Their livers and kidneys are the organs that detoxify them. Therefore, these should be eaten sparingly. I recommend the eating of brains, however, since they do not contain fat. Chicken and pork are so-called "white" meats. These should be eaten sparingly. That is, if you are healthy and want to build up into a physical marvel. If you exercise regularly, though, you need "red" meat to build up your muscles, even if you are a woman and happen to exercise less.

Second Way (Continued). The Best Meats to Eat

One of the best meats to eat is fish. Seafish, in particular. Seafoods contain iodine, which is believed to be important to the functioning of the thyroid gland. A malfunctioning thyroid gland (hyperthyroid) accelerates your heartbeat and overworks your heart. Fish alone, however, is not a particularly good blood builder, but it does build muscle, as it is a protein. Fresh-water fish is good food, but it will not do for you what salt-water fish will. It won't build up your thyroid, and you need a normally functioning thyroid gland to have a well functioning heart. Canned fish is all right, but first pour off the oil. Too much oil pads your body (and the insides of your arteries) with fat. That seems to constrict them and lead to a premature stroke. Too much oil in your stomach, too, is indigestible, overworks it and encourages acidosis. It also overworks your liver and contributes to cirrhosis. Even consuming too much oil in the natural state, as from eating too many nuts, affects you. *Warning:* Much fresh fish nowadays contain poisonous chemicals.

Yogatronics then, recommends meat of some kind as your best heavy food for supper. Meat, unless fried or cured, is comparatively easy to digest and is a filling food. It should be filling but easily digestible, or it will lie in your stomach for hours after you eat it and strain your heart, which is trying to supply enough blood to your digestive apparatus and your muscles at the same time. Your heart, remember, works 48 percent harder when digesting your food than when not digesting it.

Second Way (Continued). Eat Raw Vegetables

All through *Yogatronics*, of course, I recommend the eating of raw vegetables, with exceptions like winter squash, string beans and possibly potatoes, which, if eaten, should be baked or steamed.

Third Way to Raise Your Alpha-Cholesterol

Eat green vegetables like peas, spinach, lettuce, and especially carrots and celery because they have a high fiber content. All through *Yogatronics* I recommend these very vegetables, except spinach because of its high oxalic acid content, which robs your body of too much calcium.

Fourth Way to Raise Your Alpha-Cholsterol

Eat nearly any fresh fruit, including apples, oranges, peaches. These are all recommended by the *Yogatronic Diet*.

Fifth Way to Raise Your Alpha-Cholesterol

Dr. Wissler says *no* bananas because they have a "high fat content." I disagree with this conclusion. An ideal staying-with-you lunch dessert is the banana. It is still a fresh fruit and thus, comparatively easy to digest, but it is also heavy enough to stay with you for hours after your meal. Its sugar is not absorbed swiftly, like fructose, which is in other fruits. On the contrary, it is available to you for hours after you eat it, either at work or in sport. The banana won't constipate you like the usual sandwich, but it will not encourage loose bowels. It builds up your body weight, too, but does not fatten, and it is available most of the year. "We" find it perfect for keeping our weights ideal.

Note: The government's handbook *Composition of Foods*, lists bananas as containing .2 grams of fat compared to 13.7 for chicken, and 16.4 for turkey, yet Dr. Wissler recommends both chicken and turkey highly. A consensus of specialists in heart disease also say that potassium is essential for a healthy heart, and that a deficiency in potassium can trigger irregular heartbeats. Bananas happen to be one of the finest natural sources of potassium! The heart specialists add, furthermore, that *prolonged inactivity* can lead to excretion of potassium by the kidneys. Although I knew nothing about bio-chemistry at the age of 10, when biochemistry was hardly conceived as a science anyhow, I was still right to exercise vigorously and *systematically*, although the leading scientists of the day warned the world of the dangers of exercise and its developing a life-shortening "athlete's heart."

Sixth Way to Raise Your Alpha-Cholesterol

Avoid canned fruits packed with syrup. Fresh pineapple, watermelon, grapefruit, oranges and tomatoes, are great mucus-killing foods. To be mucus-killing when canned, however, they have to be processed without sugar. Sugared canned food is mucus-forming. Sweets also create mucus; not natural sweets, like grapes, but all foods sweetened with any concentrated sweetener, such as sugar, honey and so on. To remain in perfect health, eat a minimum of mucus-forming foods. The usual fruit salad made up of mixed canned fruits in syrup, along with diced up fresh fruits, is something to avoid. It sours your stomach and bloats you with gas. When served in restaurants, where most dishes must be prepared in quantity ahead of time, most of the vitamins and minerals are destroyed through exposure to air.

Seventh Way to Raise Your Alpha-Cholesterol

Any kind of fish is good, like trout or perch. One of the best meats to eat is fish, sea-fish, in particular.

Eighth Way to Raise Your Alpha-Cholesterol

Dr. Wissler recommends avoiding shellfish, like shrimp, lobster or crab. The *Yogatronic Diet* differs with Dr. Wissler, and states that shrimps, crabs, lobsters and scallops are very valuable in your diet, although they are on the expensive side.

I stand firm behind that statement and can prove it with the findings of science. Although, in proportion of units, shrimps contain fat (20), they also contain a fair amount of potassium, which helps the heartbeat. Scallops contain even more fat (23) but also contain considerable potassium (456). Crabs contain *very little* fat (1.6) but have no potassium. Lobster contains very little fat (1.9) and yet contains a fair amount of potassium (180). Also, for the *Yogatronic Diet* I recommend sea-weed, the only food supplement I still take, because it is no more than a dried food. It contains *5,000 to 8,000* units of potassium. Such a colossal amount of potassium can help your heart to an unbelievable degree, even if you eat shellfish. The fat in shellfish helps to fill out your face and neck and enhance your youthful appearance. *Yogatronics* also recommends the eating of much fibrous food. The fiber will absorb much of the fat of the shellfish in your intestines before it is absorbed in your blood.

Ninth Way to Raise Your Alpha-Cholesterol

Dr. Wissler states that turkey and chicken are the best fowl to eat, but limits it to the white meat because it has less fat than the dark meat. *Yogatronics* cautions, in opposition to the study, that they should be eaten sparingly.

Chickens confined all day to tiny individual coops, with their actions constricted to standing or sitting, eating a corn-mix laced with hormones and other growth-promoting supplements, cannot produce fatless white meat! Neither will white meat build muscle like lean red meat. Your heart being a muscle, it has to work harder when your other muscles are not developed enough, and tends to hypertrophy.

My Own Obvious Conclusion

Yogatronics is unquestionably an excellent producer of alpha-cholesterol. That is probably why it has been so effective with those who have followed it. It never recommends salt. There is enough natural salt in the *Yogatronic Diet*'s foods—and in sardines, too, if you wish to add them to your "wise eating." Science has proved that *Yogatronics* is ideal for high blood pressure because it consists of so many fruits and vegetables that are high in potassium and low in salt,[4] such as raw apples, bananas, avocado, cantaloupe, dates, fresh grapefruit, stewed dried apricots, cooked, dried prunes, dried raisins, fresh corn, fresh asparagus, lentils, beans, raw peas, brussel sprouts; raw, shredded cabbage, fresh cauliflower, raw green peppers, baked potatoes, raw red radishes, winter or summer squash and unsalted (unroasted) nuts and soybeans.

Yogatronics also adds a word of caution. Stewed figs, stewed dried apricots and other stewed dried fruits are all delicious and nutritious desserts. But, be sure that the dried fruit you eat has been sun-dried. Avoid those processed with sulphur-dioxide or other preservatives. All such desserts also contain sugar, but the sugar is in an organic form.

An Apple A Day Keeps High Blood Pressure Away

A Japanese researcher[5] reported in the *British Medical News* that an apple a day may keep down high blood pressure, which is linked with heart attacks. Japanese doctors experimented with Japanese workers in different regions of the country and found that on a one apple a day diet, there was a significant drop in their blood pressures. There was also a lower incidence of brain hemmorrhage among the young Japanese working in the apple-growing regions as compared to those working in other farming regions of the country.

Fresh pineapple and apples are excellent mucous-killing foods and should be made a steady part of your diet. However, I caution that apples and other fruits with coarse skins, take too long to digest because of their thick, hard skins. Always grate or shred such fruits before eating them. Even grapes with thick skins fill people with gas. Fruit skin is like the leather off the animal. When the fruit is dried, like the raisin and the prune, its skin is still hard to digest. That's why prunes and raisins should be tenderized somewhat before they are eaten. If you suffer from stomach trouble, avoid fruits with thick or leathery skins or with skins that cannot be grated down fine before putting them into the mouth. Leathery skins cause your stomach to secrete so much acid to digest them that it turns your stomach sour and fills you with gas.

Salt, I must point out, raises your blood pressure, and it is true that quite a number of the health-giving foods listed in *Yogatronics* contain salt: carrots, beets, asparagus, almonds, beans, cabbage, celery stalks, chicken leg, dandelion greens, eggs, kohlrabi, lamb, lentils, beef liver, mackerel, trout, white turnips and so on. But when salt occurs naturally in the food, it does not put weight on you. With wise eating, my wife and I keep our weights *exactly* what they were when we were at our physiological primes at 20 years of age. The record of my last boxing contest upholds this. We also exercise strenuously every day, as well as do full-time work in our careers. I seldom spend less than nine hours a day at my desk and then have a four-hour workout. It proves that the *Yogatronic Diet* must fill me with alpha-cholesterol. For many years now I have used the Triple Tonic Secret (Illus. 5, page 49) and feel as young and spry as ever.

How, Since I was 20-21, I Keep My Weight Ideal

Practically everybody I have known along the years has either gained weight as he (or she) grew older and raised his blood pressure, or has lost weight and looks much older. I weigh *exactly* what I did in my physical prime, when I fought my last boxing bout at the age of 20 years and 10 months. That's why I look almost the same year after year. I am not maintaining that same weight by losing muscle and adding fat. Neither am I atrophying, unless it is to a microscopic degree. My heart, liver, lungs, kidneys, intestines and other organs must be practically the same size they were in my youth prime. My digestive glands must be about the same, for I have the same big appetite I always had. Yet, I am not the born-to-be-thin type, as I weighed 17-1/2 pounds at birth. I also managed to gain 35 pounds when I purposely bulked up to a massive size at forty-two. In my twenties, during the poverty-starvation years that followed the loss of my small inheritance, I weighed 38 pounds below normal.

My weight, in other words, *can* fluctuate. But the *Yogatronic Diet* keeps it *exactly* what it was when I was at my physical-physiological peak at 20-21. Everybody's weight, it is true, tends to return to a "natural weight" when he eats and lives normally. With the passing years, however, the body undergoes fatty degeneration and gets heavier, or it atrophies or wastes away and weighs less. Or, it undergoes both changes at the same time and weighs the same, but is a weakened "old" body.

But I do even more and *even harder exercise* now than I did as a youth! So, my body has not undergone weakening fatty degeneration or atrophied—at least, not to an extent worth mentioning. That's why I know that I will live to over 300. I am achieving similar results with my close followers. And I am maintaining the "best weight" for the longest life I am capable of, according to the mortality investigations conducted by a number of life insurance companies, and which the Metropolitan Life Insurance Company developed, over nearly 40 years into a table. (pages 30-31).

REFERENCES

[1]Dr. William Castelli, director of laboratories for the Framington Heart Studies Research Center in Framington, Mass., who studied 2,000 people over an eight-year period, *National Enquirer*, Jan. 3, 1977.

[2]Robert W. Wissler, director of the Atherosclerosis Specialized Center of Research at the University of Chicago's Pritzker School of Medicine, *National Enquirer*, (1976-1978).

[3]*Lancet*, London, April 24, 1976.

[4]Dr. Marvin Moser, medical consultant to the National High Blood Pressure Education Program, May 25, 1976, *National Enquirer*.

[5]Dr. N. Sasski, of Japan's Hirosaki University, *National Enquirer*, July 28, 1974.

8

Yogatronic Secrets for Ideal Weight, Living Longer and Looking Younger

Science's Thoroughly Proved Seven-Year Study of How to Live Longer and Look Younger

In order to live longer and look younger, keep your weight ideal. Your waist has to remain small enough for you, and your weight light enough for you. When you neglect your waist and your weight, you invite disease, look old and shorten your life. Man has spent thousands of years searching the earth for the Fountain of Youth. He still searches desperately for that elusive secret.

A seven-year, million-dollar federally sponsored study to find the answer was conducted with 7,000 Americans.[1] The study found eight golden rules:

1. Eat regularly.
2. Don't snack between meals.
3. Eat breakfast every day.

4. Get between seven and nine hours' sleep each night.
5. Keep your weight around normal.
6. Don't smoke.
7. Have no more than 2 or 3 drinks a day.
8. Exercise regularly.

The Wonders of the Proof

Dr. Ira Cain, one of the researchers involved in the study, announced that it proved that a man of 55, who followed all the rules, possessed the same physical status as a man from 25 to 30 years younger who followed only 2 or 3 of them. The highest death risk was among the individuals who smoked more than two packs a day. Exercise, he insisted, contributed importantly to health. Men who exercised only occasionally had two times the mortaiity of men who exercised regularly. No more than two drinks a day had little effect on the lifespan. Those who ate breakfast nearly every day and did not eat between meals, had definitely better physical health than those who skipped breakfast and ate between meals.

Another researcher and coauthor of the group's report, Nedra B. Belloc, stated that it demonstrated that the daily habits of the average person had far more to do with what made him ill and how long he would live than all the influences of medicine. Men who followed the eight health habits had an 11-year increase in longevity. But the life expectancy of American men of 45 had lengthened, between 1900 and 1970, *no more than* 3 years, despite all the advances of modern medicine. Avoiding bad habits and adopting good ones, the coauthor concluded, could lead to a long healthy existence.

The researchers also found that being underweight is just as unhealthy as being overweight. Individuals who were 10 per cent or more underweight had the highest mortality rate. When people passed 20 per cent overweight their mortality rate increased rapidly.

The Miracle of Yogatronics

Metabolically speaking, you ought to remain no more than thirty practically all your life.

In the last twenty-three years, I have improved the now scientifically proven *Yogatronic Diet* and reaped such fantastic results with it, that I have increased my longevity expectation to at least 300, and yet to look no more than 50. And I expect to do so while still living in big polluted cities and eating devitalized, insecticide-sprayed food!

Here are the amazing detailed revelations of the *Yogatronic Diet* for ideal weight, living longer and looking younger, arranged in the order of the "golden rules" of the report.

Golden Rules 1 and 2: *"Eat regularly, and don't snack between meals."*

Yogatronics advises three meals a day, consumed at the same time every day. This is an unshakable rule for a trim body and small waist, because all of Nature works with regularity. The lunch hour alone can be shifted now and then, without ill effects. But try *never* to shift breakfast or supper time, because shifting them only upsets the regularity of your system. You can alter your lunch time now and then, if you can't avoid it, but eat your heavy meals at regular times. By doing so, you fill your stomach at regular times and induce digestion and peristaltic action at regular times. Eating with regularity is an important contributor to lifetime health and eternal youth.

Regularity also trains your digestive system to expect anxiously to be fed at a certain hour. Precisely at that hour, the glands start secreting slightly, even if no food is put in your stomach. If you eat right then, you catch your stomach at its *digestive prime*.

Furthermore, your tissues, at a precise time after this, are best ready to absorb the right amount of food which your body needs. At that time they won't be overfed or starved. You are less likely to overeat or undereat.

Regularity also improves your appetite, since you feed yourself at the best time possible. This is another reason why *Yogatronics* opposes fasting. By denying your body the food it craves—expecially at the very time it craves it most—you torture it and develop in it an instinctive fury against all food restrictions. When you get off the fast, your vengeance-seeking appetite goes berserk and drives you to gobble up gluttonous portions of the worst foods. Shortly after the fast, therefore, your system could be in the worst shape it has ever been in and could dread, thereafter, the very suggestion of a fast or a diet.

Golden Rules 1 and 2 (Continued)

Rhythm regularity, your body's unmatchable weight-regulator. Yogatronics discloses the secret of Rhythm Regularity, also called Bio-rhythm by science. Rhythm Regularity is the body's weight-regulator, which must be developed and kept working for you. The word diet is misleading. Diet suggests the starving and limiting of your natural appetite. *Yogatronics* is against curbing your appetite through any method whatsoever—unless you do so under a doctor's orders. Curbing it—especially by swallowing substances which cut down appetite, fool your taste glands, so that they lose much of their ability to let you know what particular foods your system needs most. As a result, you lose weight and, perhaps, your health, too.

Meal-time regularity spins into action a Rhythm Regularity in your whole system—a regularity of prime importance in bringing you a long-lasting life, saturated with the joys of good health.

Rhythm Regularity trains your body to respond most intensely to food at *specific times* during the day, or to the specific times you eat your three square meals. A wave of appetite rushes upon you at these times and enables your body to extract the utmost nutriment out of your food. That's why I have been able to maintain amazing health on depleted, devitalized supermarket and city grocery food all these decades and feel healthy enough to live another 300 years.

The Magic Power of Rhythm Regularity

In an extensive study involving a total of over 5,000 analyses, Arnold Osterberg and his co-researchers[2] discovered that about 80 percent of the subjects produced "normal" values of the digestive enzyme *pepsin* in the "test tube" meal. These "normal" values ranged between 0 for some, up to 449 units for others. About 20 percent of the values were above "normal," most of them yielding from 1000 to 1999 units and a very small number of them yielding over 2000 units. None of these individuals exhibited any signs of gastric disease. The total range between all of them was an extraordinary 0 to 4300 units.

When you train yourself to eat with Rhythm Regularity you catch your stomach, at mealtime, at its digestive prime. Instead of secreting a minor amount of gastric juice, digesting your food only partially and letting much of its depleted vitamins and minerals pass out unabsorbed, you absorb them to the maximum degree that can amount to as much as 4300 times what other "normal" people would absorb out of it. Even in your own body, it could amount to many times your own "normal" absorption. This grows more important the older you become, when your stomach secretes less gastric juice. Since the concentration of gastric juice varies significantly with your frame of mind, with Rhythm Regularity you can train it to secrete such an overwhelming amount of gastric juice, at any point in life, that your digestion potential never ages. You likewise absorb the utmost benefit out of your food all your life. With Rhythm Regularity you can extract so much more nutriment out of your commercialized, depleted food that you won't need food supplements. And if you do take supplements, you can take far less of them, because your stomach would absorb far more out of them. Otherwise, you may be excreting too much of them unabsorbed and chronically irritating your liver, kidneys and bladder.

A healthy flood of gastric juice empties your digestive glands at each meal, and you will hardly be hungry between meals and need snacks.

Golden Rule 3.

Eat breakfast every day. SOLAR DIET already advised you to have "three meals a day." Three meals a day consist of breakfast, lunch and supper.

Golden Rule 4

Get between seven and nine hours sleep every night. To bulk up for body building you ought to sleep eight hours a night, providing that you rest twice during the day, a half hour or less each time; otherwise, you should sleep for nine hours. If you are not bulking up, you should obviously rest less, which would total to around eight hours.

Golden Rule 5

Keep your weight always ideal. (One out of five American men, and one out of four women, are 10 percent or more overweight). *Yogatronics* holds that in order to gain beneficial weight, you cannot ignore the laws of health. Health is the primary goal of all diet or exercise. It is possible to gain weight without ruining your body or your health. But to do so, stick closely to natural means. Your basic diet should remain the same, and you should still follow the general rules of the *Yogatronic Diet*. And remember this! *Don't try* to gain or lose all your weight overnight. Everyone has his own natural metabolic rate, and to interfere with it is to flirt with disaster. You are advised, in brief, to gain weight only if it is normal for you to do so, and to do it by natural means.

In other words, *Yogatronics* teaches you how to retain your healthiest weight, and the scientific study proves that your healthiest weight is your ideal weight. The *Yogatronic Diet* goes even further and shows you the safe way to retain it.

Golden Rule 6

Don't smoke. The *Yogatronic Diet* states that smoking between meals, or in fact at any time, is not recommended.

Golden Rule 7

Don't have more than two or three drinks a day. Yogatronics recommends *no liquor.* If 1 or 3 are the most drinks you should take, according to the study, taking 1 or none should be better still. Liquor of any kind is a stomach acidifier.

Neither *eat* nor *drink* before going to bed. Don't drink even a fruit or vegetable juice.

Abstain from eating or drinking late at night. After a show, don't stop in a restaurant for a late supper or in the drug store for an ice cream or malted milk. Don't take a drink, either alcoholic or soft, between supper and bedtime either.

Social life, it is true, is composed of these little amenities. Friends and associates "drop into" places after going out together or running into each other, in order to sit and chat a little. To refuse to join your friends in a "bite" or a "refreshment" is to create hard feelings or to pass for a food crank.

But you don't have to refuse them outright. Go along with them to the places, but tell them that you will only sip water because nothing else agrees with you after supper. Don't beat around the bush and tell them that you don't like beer or malted milk. If it bothers you not to order with the others, order the beverage anyway, but sip only from the glass of water that is served with it. If you fear it would limit your social life, select foods that are easiest to digest (like fruits and unseasoned vegetables), and before breakfast neutralize your over-acidified stomach with two glasses of unsweetened pineapple juice.

Golden Rule 8

Exercise regularly. I wrote physical fitness courses as early as 1960, and followed them with hard-cover books like YOGA FOR MEN ONLY, SOMO-PSYCHIC POWER and YOGA SECRETS FOR EXTRAORDINARY HEALTH AND LONG LIFE.[3]

All were published from 1 to 11 years before the scientific study revealed its golden rules. All of them taught my students and readers to exercise regularly. I have been exercising regularly and systematically from the age of 10, despite the dire warnings of the scientists of that day.

Now I'll provide you with the most advanced *Yogatronic Diet* exercise magic rule, another one which science probably won't discover for a long, long time.

There is Little Reason Why You Can't Live to 300

There is nothing incredible about living long and being youthful and trim, with a small waist and an active mind. Don't worry about your kidneys, your liver, your stomach, your colon or intestines. According to science, your kidneys can function to 150 years. You have two of them, which extends their total lifespan to 300 years. Your liver has "indefinite" reserves in unused tissue. You don't have to smoke and shortchange your lungs. Hence, they can last seemingly forever. Big city pollution does not devastate them as speedily as some scientists believe. It has not affected my lungs or my wife's.

For about 2 years, between the ages of 29-31, I was in such desperate circumstances that I worked in a factory in which undiluted benzene was used all day long to wash paint off of glass. Benzene exposure has been linked to leukemia and a federal safety standard will limit worker's exposure to 1 part of benzene per 1,000,000 parts of air. The Environmental Protection Agency even lists *public* exposure to it as hazardous, which is considerably less than that of the workers. Yet my lungs are in wonderful shape and I do not suffer from leukemia. I *do not support* any kind of pollution. I am just giving you the factual proofs of the survival of your organs and making you realize that you shouldn't look hopelessly to the future and expect a severely shortened life, just because you didn't grow up living in a Shangri-la like Hunza, Maracaibo or the Caucasus. I will reveal the secret at the end of this chapter.

THE TWO WEAK POINTS THAT RUIN YOUR FIGURE AND SHORTEN YOUR LIFE

(1) Your first weak spot is your *arteries*, your coronary arteries, in particular. When they are narrowed by cholesterol plaques, (atherosclerosis), or their walls are hardened by fibrous tissue (arterosclerosis) you are on the road to senility and to the loss of a clear mind. Either of these conditions, even to a slight degree, reduces your muscular and mental activities and fattens your body and your waist. They rob you of youth and trimness, raise your blood pressure and doom you to be classified among the aging no matter how young you may be.

(2) Your second weak spot is your joints. Unfortunately, they may be ruined by the very activities you engage in to acquire your trim body and small waist. Among these are jogging, tennis, handball, weight-lifting, rope-skipping, hiking, baseball, basketball, bicycling and many others. Your knees and ankles—your knees, expecially—are the joints that degenerate from the micro-trauma of overuse into osteoarthritis. With the passing years, they wear down and leave you stiff-legged and aching. Your hip-joint is another vulnerable joint. Since no plastic joint equals a normal one, I gave up jogging 23 years ago, in favor of a better exercise. Now, 23 years later, science lauds jogging. Eventually, I predict, it will agree with me about the greater value of the much better miracle exercise I discovered and which I describe next.

My Miracle Discovery Beyond Jogging

The first advance discovery I made beyond jogging was top speed sprinting for short distances, interrupted by walking two or three times that short distance. With sprinting, I have been accelerating my heartbeat and breathing much faster than with jogging, and I spare my ankles and knees from thousands of needless traumatic steps. In my book, YOGA SECRETS FOR EXTRAORDINARY HEALTH AND LONG LIFE, I discussed at length, my insistence that sprinting does more for the heart than jogging, and prophesied that science will prove me right. Now, I have discovered a still better way. The list which follows classifies exercise in increasing order of calorie consumption.[4]

Exercise

Light exercise

Walking slowly (2.6 miles per hour)

Active exercise

Walking moderately fast (3.7 miles per hr.)

Severe exercise

Swimming
Running (5.3 mi. per hr.)

Very severe exercise

Walking very fast (5.3 mi. per hr.)
Walking up stairs.

Walking up stairs expends nearly 2½ times the amount of energy as *severe exercise*, expending over twice that of swimming or running.

Science Upholds My Miracle Discovery

No test has been made, apparently, on anyone sprinting up steep stairs by twos. But it obviously requires a tremendous amount of energy. That of jogging, in comparison to it, would be child's play. Such an exercise would bring you the strongest heart you could probably develop—and do it in a fraction of the time of jogging or the other exercises measured. Your knees, ankles and other joints would be spared immeasurably. You would no longer have to watch everything you eat "like a hawk," because you would use up so much energy.

If you are in sound health, start by climbing two or three flights by twos very fast. Do so five times a week. Don't climb steps in high heels or cramping shoes, but use comfortable, low-heeled shoes. Don't hang on to the bannister, but swing your bent arms back and forth alternately, like a sprinter, and throw your whole body into the effort. As the weeks go by, push your body higher in the air at each step with the balls of your feet. *That* is when you sprint. Your heart will be pounding full blast by the time you reach the top stairs. If you live in a high-rise, gradually add more flights of stairs to your workout. Your thighs will turn firm and shapely, and your heart and lungs phenomenally stronger. I find twelve flights at one time, once a day, to be the peak exercise necessary for top condition. Your body will stay trim and youthful, and your waist will remain small. Your heart and lungs will last "forever."

The Triple Tonic Secret for "Ideal Weight," Living Longer and Looking Younger

Beyond the eight rules, the Triple Tonic Secret can add to your health. It took hold of my body like a vise, squeezed my waist even smaller and filled my movements with an acrobatic lightness that made me feel and look another ten years younger. Here is its secret. (Follow Illus. 10).

1. Blast the odic force from your intermediate lobe to sides of your torso (Illus. 10A).
2. With it, force the odic force of your torso off of your torso, and "rip off" your torso fat.
3. Blast the odic force from your intermediate lobe to the front of your abdomen (Illus. 10B).
4. With it, force the odic force off your abdomen, and "rip off" your abdominal fat.

How Ramsay B. Seemed to have Become Immortal

I had known Ramsay B. slightly, twenty-five years before on the beach, but had not seen him since. He reappeared on the beach one day—looking only a *little older* and *much trimmer*. When I expressed stark surprise and praised his secret whatever it was, he told me that it could be no secret to me because it was *my* secret that he had followed. He had overheard me, twenty-five years ago, describing to a body builder exactly how to eat, to take the best care of oneself. I had impressed him so much with it, Ramsay said, that after he went home, he jotted down all of it he remembered. "It beat anything about nutrition I had read any-

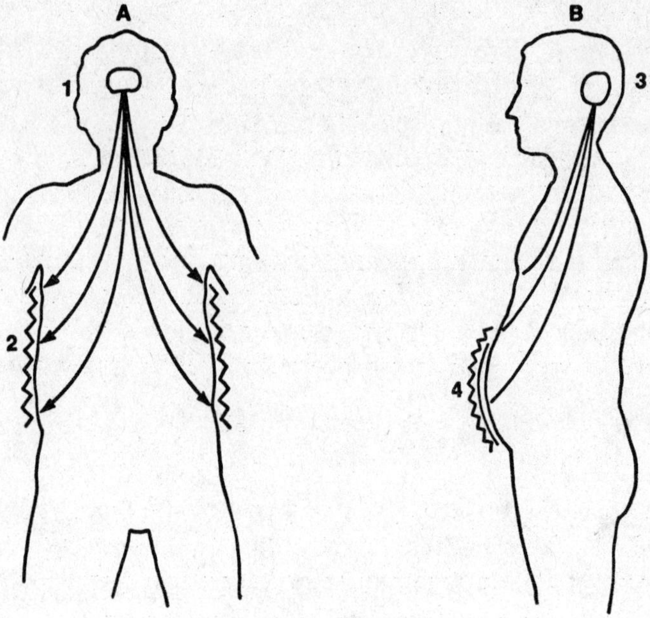

Illustration 10

where," he told me. "It worked miracles with me, as you can very well see!" He had overheard only a sample of what I published in SOLAR DIET two years later. Ramsay was eager to add to it the secrets of the *Yogatronic Diet* and now aims to live to be 300 years old himself.

How Betty-Lou H. Bid Good-Bye to her Needless Fat and Stiffening Joints

Betty-Lou H., like so many other people, searched for decades for a daily way of life that would slenderize her, lengthen her life, and also make her look comparatively young. Too many people she knew, she moaned, lived "frightful lives" after middle-age. They had been "abandoned by the world" because they had "lost their shapes" or "looked old and drifted around with one foot in the grave."

I disclosed to Betty-Lou the very same *Yogatronic Diet* rules of eating which science has incorporated into eight golden rules for providing a person, at 55, with the physical status of someone 25 to 30 years younger who follows only 2 to 5 of them. In ten or eleven weeks, by following them, Betty-Lou underwent an astounding transformation. Then she added the ninth golden rule of *Yogat-*

ronic Diet to them. She lost 35 lbs. and looked fifteen years younger. She felt so light and limber that she took up tennis and soon played a fine game.

THE MAGIC FOOD THAT PROTECTS YOU FROM THE RAVAGES OF POLLUTION

Although I have lived four-fifths of my life in three of the most polluted metropoles of the world, as I have stated several times before, I am in perfect health. My lungs, my blood and the rest of my body have escaped intact. Without suspecting why, I have found out now that I owe much to the wonder food garlic. Experiments in Japan and Russia prove that garlic collects lead, mercury, cadmium and other toxic metals in your body and excretes them in your bowels. (This is due obviously, to the sulphydryl radical which I tracked down and described thoroughly before). A doctor in *Runner's World*, after learning of these discoveries, suggests to joggers who breathe the poisonous exhausts of traffic to take garlic to "stay healthy." Other researchers found that garlic is also effective in treating anemia, arthritis, diabetes and far more dangerous body conditions. But it had to be fresh garlic, they insisted. You could not use processed garlic powder and garlic salt as a substitute, for these had lost too much of their potencies.

I had already taught all these discoveries to my students in *Solar Diet*, twenty-five years before science. I did not suspect then that garlic combined also with the heavy metals of the polluted air, but my students and I gained from that life-prolonging advantage nonetheless by following my advice to the letter, including eating fresh garlic rather than processed garlic.

Let me add that I disagree, however, with the researchers who find garlic effective in treating anemia. Since garlic and onions help prevent blood clots they are obviously blood thinners, not blood thickeners.

REFERENCES

[1]The study began in 1965, and was funded by the National Center for Health Services Research and Development.

[2]Arnold E. Osterberg, Frances R. Vanzanto, Walter C. Alvarez, and Andrew B. Rivera, *Am. J. Digestive Diseases*, 3, 35-41, 1936.

[3]All books by Parker Publishing Company, Inc., West Nyack, New York.

[4]Compiled by M.S. Rose, from Sherman, H. C.: *Chemistry of Food and Nutrition*, New York, 1941. The Macmillan Co.

9

How Yogatronics Banishes Energy-Wasting Weight

The Telling Taste-Crave

Good nutrition is most important to perfect the wisdom of your body to select the right food and the right amount you should eat. You are guided otherwise by the unhealthy food tastes you cultivate and ruin your trimness and your waist (and your internal organs and other parts of you). You ought to speedily restrict or terminate a craving for refined sugar or its products, or it will confuse your natural taste and ruin the benefits of your diet.

The belief that one food feeds you better than another, is not held by *Yogatronics*. Not enough is known about all vitamins and minerals to enable anyone to positively declare that one live food is better than another. The only reliable guide, so far, is *which live food you crave most*. That food is the one which you probably need most. Your natural appetite reaches out for the nutrition which your body requires most and thereby keeps your weight close to your own natural body weight. In an experiment on nutrition, Dr. Susan Lustick from Cornell University, who teaches at Michael Reese Hospital School of Nursing, Chicago, discovered that no matter how she starved or tried to fatten her subjects, once the attempt ceased, they either went back up or down to their own natural weight. This weight-maintenance is apparently controlled by the hypothalamus. Your natural appetite reaches out for the nutrition which your body requires most. The missing nutrition in your body, in some way, alters the craving in your taste glands—a craving which is satisfied *only* when you taste food containing the missing nutrition. A calcium or mineral-starved baby will swallow chalk or soil because its taste glands react to the taste or mineral present in the chalk or soil. This taste-crave (except when applied to sweets, condiments and other health-ruining foods) is Nature's best guide to help you select the foods which your body needs most. This eating guide of yours must also be controlled by your appestat, the primitive eating center concealed in your hypothalamus.

The Shape-Ruining Addiction

It is difficult for the usual test to discover what nutrition your body is most in need of. The efficacy of the test, for one thing, is limited by the extent of the knowledge held by man, at the moment, about food. Thirty years ago, about five or six vitamins were known. In another thirty years, heaven knows how many more will be found. The way they are combined, too, might have much to do with their effectiveness. Besides, the foods that are praised because they contain the vitamins known today, might be considered inadequate thirty years from now because they might not contain enough of the vitamins discovered by then; while, the foods that are condemned today might be held in the highest esteem thirty years from now. That is exactly what is occurring even now. The world is finally accepting garlic as a health saver, drinking many glasses of water daily, eating bulk foods and raw foods and is discarding spinach, cod-liver oil and much cooked food. Such alternating repudiation and acceptance will go on until Judgment Day.

In following the lead of your taste craving, which you will learn how to dominate at the end of this chapter with the Triple Tonic Secret for it, beware of developing a gluttonous appetite for the food elements you *already* have, and sadly deprive yourself of those you need. You can stuff yourself with cake and ice cream, for instance, *long after* your daily need for sugar is satisfied. A test panel discovered that sugar becomes an *addiction*, that the body or the psyche finds something actually voluptuous or ecstatic in the sweet taste. Sweets are like opiates, the scientists went on, in that they control behavior powerfully. People of all cultures, in the past as well as present, have been ready to do anything to eat large amounts of sugar.[1] Your taste for sugar, in brief, can be developed far beyond your natural need for sugar.

In another study, rats were given a choice between nutritional foods and sugar-water. The rats drank the sugar-water and bypassed the food until they died of malnutrition. No wonder science warns you not to get started on the *sugar habit*, and calls it the "sugar connection with a psychological addiction."

The Missing Freeing Element

Your taste glands alone, then, cannot—and will not—balance your body needs accurately. You *still need* a balanced diet. You need, in short, both the foods which your body craves, as well as an expertly balanced diet, supplemented with the best proper combinations of vitamins and minerals known. I have found that the Triple Tonic Secret is the best food supplement a man can have. I have proved it by continuing to live in big polluted cities, eating the depleted foods sold in them and being constantly subjected to endless environmental tensions. It is conceivable that you could do much better with both the ideal food from the ground and living in a small, quiet, ideal community. But, since that is an impossible dream for most of us, it is reassuring to learn that you *can* fare just about as well right where you are, with wise eating and by adding the Triple Tonic Secret to your meals.

Your Sadly Lost Body Wisdom

When your diet is deficient, particularly in thiamine (vitamin B_1), your body loses its "wise food" selection wisdom.[2] You lose your appetite and starve yourself. In experiments with animals on a deficient diet, all lost their food-selection wisdom, consuming high levels of alcohol and ignoring nourishing food. In contrast, when fed nourishing food only, they shunned alcohol. Their body wisdom told them *what* to shun to stay healthy. Some shunned alcohol less than others, because their requirements for certain items of diet were higher and therefore harder to satisfy. The same principle held true with respect to sugar consumption.[3] Rats fed on deficient diets chose to eat more sugar than rats fed on nutritious food. *First*, the scientists concluded, it proves that food deficiencies too mild to cause diagnosable lesions significantly lower the wisdom of food selection in individual animals. *Second*, it proves that the animals needed substances in food which were *not* recognized by man, to enable them to develop maximum food-selection widom. *Third*, it proves that you, like everybody else, possess your own individual distinctive pattern of food needs. *Fourth*, it proves that important deficiencies in your body may exist which elude diagnosis.

Long before science knew about carbohydrates, fats, proteins, minerals and vitamins, people who lived close to the soil consumed these nutrients in generally the right proportions, and large numbers of these people did not suffer from the symptoms of deficient nutrition. Today, with all the counts against the food you eat, *few* people escape malnutrition—even the so-called "well-fed." Most people have actually lost their primitive taste-crave, the power of their body wisdom to select the right food for them to eat. Misleading advertising, food-oriented social life and countless other enemies of a proper diet make matters even worse.

How to Regain Your Lost Body Wisdom

For years now, with the *Yogatronic Diet* I have been taking two most important steps to regain my body wisdom.

1. I eat foods that apparently counteract, to a most effective degree, the massive amounts of poisons which I swallow daily in the food from my big city supermarket or corner grocery.

2. I pile-drive my depleted meals as they digest with three blasts of the Triple Tonic Secret.

Many other people resort to vitamin-mineral supplements. I stopped recommending them five years after *Solar Diet* was published. People usually take staggering doses, forcing their bodies to secrete the excess through the kidneys and bladder. Such overconcentrations, I fear, may overirritate the mucous membranes lining their inner cavities.

For example, since the zinc content of your blood may vary

from that of other normal persons by as much as 13-fold and the calcium content can vary by as much as 4.5-fold, the scientific conclusion is that individual needs for proteins and specific amino acids must also vary substantially.[4] Even the "enhancement of intelligence" was tested in experimental animals and in mentally deficient children by administering them glutamic acid. Glutamic acid had never been considered an essential amino acid for mammals. The effects on their intelligence was conflicting, but glutamic acid did enhance the growth of weaning rats. The scientists concluded that "the subject of the effects of glutamic acid on intelligence" required to be investigated fully. In brief, it *might* or *might not* improve the intelligence.

It is absolutely impossible, as a consequence, to supply you or anyone else with a close approximation of how much of any nutrient you need. If you take in too much of it regularly, you overburden the important organs of your body like your liver, kidneys and bladder, and you hasten their degeneration. If you take in too *little* of it regularly, you bring on or retain the symptoms (even if subclinical) of its deficiencies. Yet, the need for that nutrient between you and your normal neighbor can differ by as much as 13-fold. It varies still more at specific times because of your altering biorhythms and different astrological aspects.

The Miracle Triple Tonic Secret

Food supplements, therefore, are not the unquestionable solutions to proper nutrition. The fact that they contain many times the daily requirement of any nutrient increases the possibilities of your ingesting too much of them. That's why, in the *Yogatronic Diet*, I chose to develop my body's wisdom for wise eating with the Triple Tonic Secret instead. Day by day I could sense my tissues requiring different nutrients, calibrating my telling taste-crave to hunger for the precise quantities my body needed of each. As far back as 1941 P. T. Young, E. M. Scott and others wrote extensively in journals that the wisdom of the body to eat was one of the fundamental "wisdoms of the body." My own body wisdom is apparently incredibly exact, for it has permitted me to consume big meals all my life (except during my several years of abject poverty) yet I have kept my weight the same to the very pound. Roger J. Williams calls this ability "a wisdom of the body." It was not mere chance that I have such body wisdom, because many in my family have become overweight and shortened their lives. It is not because of my hypothalamus, because I am known for possessing a voracious appetite. It was undoubtedly because of the Triple Tonic Secret, which I have always carried in my mind, even though I did not realize it until fifteen years ago. Other people may have to develop theirs, because Roger Williams himself states that the body's wisdom is not infallible in all individuals. But you *can* make it infallible, as I made mine. Learn how to choose the right foods and how much of each to eat, and banish the worthless foods. Learn how to psychically intensify the wisdom of your body to eat wisely. Follow the instructions which follow, with Illustration 11.

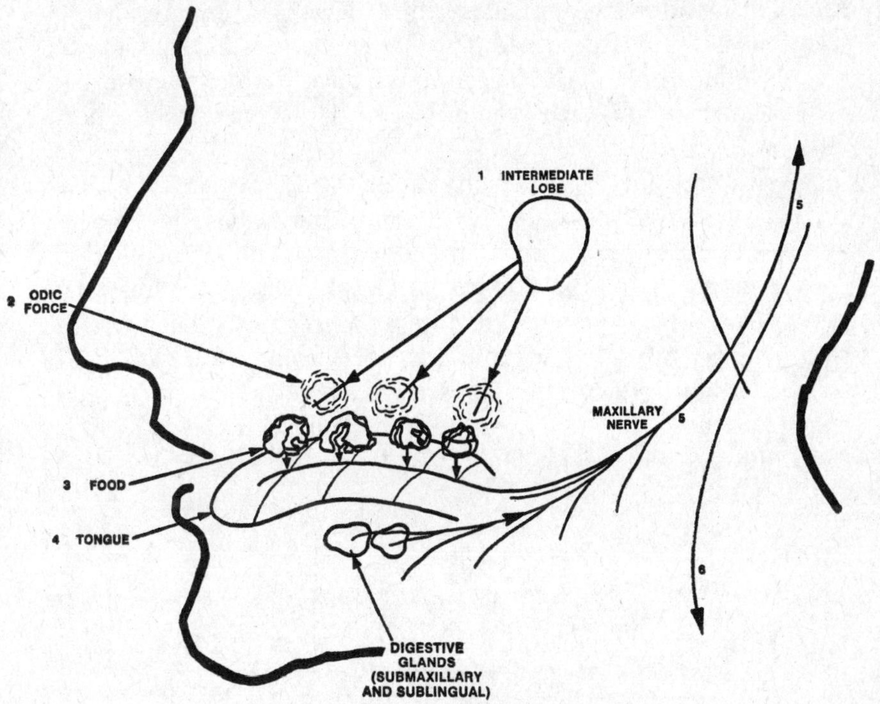

Illustration 11

1. Blast the odic force of your intermediate lobe
2. Into the odie force of the food in your mouth
3. Pressing against your tongue.
4. Drive that odic force into your nerve of taste, your lingual nerve, which innervates a good part of your tongue.

The taste of your food, after you do this during several meals, will be intensified many times.

5. Whatever nutrients your body needs will be made most emphatic to your brain.
6. Flash it to your stomach, and it will crave for these body needs and extract *far more* of them from your food than it would normally.

Percy B. Felt as if His Mind was Rejuvenated

Percy B. was 80 pounds overweight and continued eating voraciously whatever satisfied his appetite. He felt lethargic most of the time. Whenever a difficult problem confronted him at work, his mind found refuge in fantasy thinking of a juvenile sexual nature. His psychiatrist assured him that he was normal, but advised him to reduce his weight. The mind, I have frequently observed, flees frequently into sexual fantasy to escape facing wracking problems.

With the *Yogatronic Diet*, Percy started regaining his lost body wisdom swiftly and enjoying nourishing foods. Aided by the Triple Tonic Secret, he gradually added more nutritious foods to his diet and avoided the others. In a few weeks, his telling taste-crave changed so completely that he *preferred* nutritious food. His overweight diminished without his even being aware of it. He relished solving difficult problems at work and was soon assigned to special duties which could lead to remarkable advancement in his corporation.

REFERENCES

[1]Michael B. Canton, of Columbia University, and Richard J. Eichler at the City University in New York, psychologists, in the publication of the American Chemical Society. 1977.

[2]Icie G. Macy, *Nutrition and Chemical Growth in Childhood,* Charles C. Thmoas, Springfield, Il., and Baltimore, Md., Vol. 1, 1942.

[3]Roger J. Williams, Richard B. Pelton, and Lorene L. Rogers, *Quart. J. Studies Alc.*, 16, 1955. p. 234-44.

[4]*Biochemical Individuality: The Basis for the Genetotrophic Concept.* R. J. Williams, The University of Texas at Austin. Austin and London, Fifth printing. 1975.

10

yogatronics–key to warding off the effects of food poisons

FIVE SECRETS TO PROTECT YOU AGAINST COMMERCIALLY ADDED POISONS IN YOUR FOOD

As I stated before, I have lived for over half a century in the biggest, most polluted cities in America and have consumed food daily, which has been saturated with the countless chemicals, insecticides and other toxins added to them. I still drink from eight to 12 glasses daily of their chlorinated, chemically-treated water and breathe their smoggy, lung-destroying air. Yet, I am in prime health and doubt if I could be healthier had I lived in Hunza or some other earthly paradise. I probably would be in the same condition even if I lived on a small farm and raised my own food organically. My body would have had a minimum of toxins to combat, but with *Yogatronics* wise eating I reduced the maximum poisons of big city food and environment to a minimum. Let's start with the first of the five secrets to protect you from added poisons in your food.

Secret 1. The Vitamin That Nullifies the Effects of Added Food Toxins

An important nullifier of the sprays and other commercially added toxins to your food, which researchers recommend, is to regularly take an abnormal supply of vitamin C. Vitamin C can prevent the toxic effects of cyanide in coli bacteria, of phenol in rats and of lockjaw in mice, by reducing the hydrogen content of the toxins. Laboratory tests conducted by the Cancer Research Center of British Columbia in Vancouver, Canada, prove that vitamin C is virtually 100 percent effective in preventing the dreaded possible long-term pathologies of common meat preservatives. Vitamin C, announced Dr. Robert Whiting, the research chemist, blocks the potentially harmful effect of the nitrites in them. The nitrites, otherwise, combine with the hydrochloric acid in your stomach to produce nitrosamines, a dangerous product. Fifty or 100 milligrams of vitamin C, or the amount in an average orange, is enough to do the trick.[1] The vitamin should be taken at the same time as the food with the nitrite preservative.

Yogatronics has apparently saved me and my followers from the potentially ravaging effects of the insecticides in meat. I have never recommended vitamin C pills, because I find them corrosive to the lining of the bladder and perhaps to that of the kidneys as well. But the *Yogatronic Diet* includes a mass of vitamin C-containing foods like fruits or salads, to be consumed *at the same meal* with meat. In the morning it even "prescribes" the drinking of a glass of warm water containing the juice of half a lemon shortly after you get up. Lemon juice contains much vitamin C.

Studies on humans at the University of Toronto[2] upheld the results of the Cancer Research Center. In another experiement, these studies found that bran flakes were effective against abnormal cell changes caused by the nitrites. Bran flakes, I offer in explanation, have a heavy fibrous content which apparently absorbs the nitrites released in the stomach and carries them out of the body with them.

Yogatronics' natural nullifier of added food toxins

I still prefer to rely on natural sources for my vitamin C, such as vegetables and fruits. *All-bran* cereals can be too rough for the system and have been stripped of food elements.

According to the FDA *Consumer*[3], the best natural sources for vitamin C are vegetables and fruits. These are, in descending order of their concentration of the vitamin: oranges, cantaloupes, fresh orange juice, grapefruits, fresh strawberries, broccoli, spinach and other "greens," sweet potatoes, raw cabbage, white potatoes, and tomato juice. All these provide more than 20 milligrams per serving, or from one-third to half of the daily requirement recommended by the FDA. The *Yogatronic Diet* recommends all these foods for regular consumption, except spinach because of its heavy content of oxalic acid.

To continue with the government article, "Ascorbic acid (vitamin C) varies widely in fruits. Apples, apricots, peaches, pears, and prunes contain only small amounts per serving. Half a cantaloupe provides about twice as much as a wedge of watermelon. Strawberries are more than twice as rich per serving as blackberries or raspberries. Orange juice supplies about five times as much as the same amount of pineapple juice. Among the foods that provide little or no ascorbic acid (vitamin C) are dry beans, poultry, eggs, cheese, cereals, fats, oils and sugar.

"Actually, there is no way of knowing the exact ascorbic value of any particular food at the time it is eaten. Its content is affected by many factors, none of which you can really control. However, anyone who eats a sufficient number of foods known to be high in vitamin C will have no trouble obtaining the recommended amount."

The possible unforeseen consequences of taking supplements

According to all studies documented at the present time, the FDA *Consumer* continues, the body uses only the amount of ascorbic acid it needs, and eliminates the rest through the kidneys. When the body tissues are depleted in vitamin C, however, a high intake is absorbed and retained. The trouble is that your body, in a normal civilized environment, is never depleted of vitamin C. However, there is no way of determining simply how near to depletion it is because, the FDA publication stated, "There is no way of knowing the exact ascorbic value of any particular food at the time it is eaten. This is affected," the report added, "by many factors, such as conditions under which the food is grown, the time and temperature involved in handling, the kind and amount of processing or cooking it has undergone, and the conditions of storage before use." That explains why vitamin supplements are recommended by different people. The *exact* or approximate doses which you or anybody else needs at any particular time, nonetheless, are impossible to determine, and the high doses recommended for regular consumption may lead to inexplicable side effects which are difficult to foresee. The body and its tissues respond in unforeseen ways, after years or decades of exposure, to irritations which may seem minor at the time. That is why I gave up taking vitamin-mineral supplements after six years and confidently depend on natural food and The Triple Tonic Secret to supply an adequate amount.

Secret 2. The Food Toxin-Absorbing Foods That Protect You

Another, somewhat better known, way to protect you against the commercially added poisons in your food encourages the eating of fibrous foods regularly. The *Yogatronic Diet* also encourages fiber content in the diet. By keeping your digesting food moving along at a normal pace (aided by your drinking water regularly and doing the Abdominal Double Curl exercise, as shown on page 61), you will not allow it to stagnate in your alimentary tract after its nutrients are absorbed. Fiber holds water, and it also sweeps the heavy metal sprays on the food along with it, which contain mercury, arsenic and so forth. Researchers warn you not to consume *too much* fibrous food, because it will rob your body of trace minerals by carrying them out from your digesting food.

Secret 3. The Food Toxin-Reducing Drink

Milk is an effective absorber of toxins and is given to people who have swallowed poison. *Yogatronics* recommends two glasses of skim milk at breakfast and two glasses at supper.

Secret 4. The Food Toxin-Extracting Foods

You may not be familiar with the organic chemistry word *mercaptan.* A mercaptan is a chemical compound which forms insoluble mercury salts. Most remarkable, it combines with arsenic and mercury compounds *right in your cells* to form insoluble salts. It competes with your cells for the heavy metals that are brought to them by your chemically treated food. Mercaptans extract these metals from your cells and combine with them in insoluble salts which you excrete. During World War II, 2-3-dimercaptopropanol (a mercaptan) was developed as an antidote to arsenic and mercury poisoning.

Oils of garlic and onions are sulfides, and sulfides can be converted to mercaptans by the chemical action of methyl halide (C_2H_5) on them. A methyl iodide salt is such a halide, and garlic contains iodine, perhaps in the form of such an iodide salt. A chemical action between these two salts is most likely when the garlic is digested, which converts the garlic into a mercaptan. This must be a fact because *methyl mercaptan* has an odor reminiscent of garlic and onions and other "noxious" smelling substances. *Each chemical substance has its own individual unmistakable odor*! Science has apparently not discovered that such a chemical reaction takes place in garlic and converts it into a mercaptan, because the allyl radical ($-C_3H_5$) which is present in garlic, has not yet been isolated as such.[4] A mercaptan, however, contains the biochemical -SH group, which means that it is a hydrogen sulfide salt which combines with the heavy metals in your cells.

The incomparable health keeper

To the heavy dish, add garlic and onions whenever possible. Garlic is the natural, germ-killing and blood-purifying food. Blood-purifying would include the removing of food-toxins from the blood.

Eating fresh garlic and onions with the wrong food combination tremendously lessens any over-acidity that might form. Food-toxins also form over-acidity in your blood. If garlic lessens over-acidity from wrong food combinations, it can also lessen it from any other cause, such as from sprays, insecticides, etc.

Secret 5. The Food Toxin-Exterminating Triple Tonic Secrets

Every day your body goes through hours of changing susceptibilities to bacteria and infection, to anesthetics, alcohol and stimulants and to rhythms in pain tolerance. There is a variation in the production of kidney and liver enzymes and of self-regulating hormones and an excitation of allergic reaction and drug response.

Within the compass of a day there are rhythms within you for the formation of proteins. Even the keenness of your nerves probably alters in a circadian rhythm.[5] It is all proof that you *can* change your body's defensive reaction to food-toxins, for it varies daily to begin with. You can change it so that your cells refuse to absorb *any* food toxins. You may not succeed entirely, but you will leave far less of the commercially added food toxins, for the first four secrets to protect you against. You can protect yourself so effectively against food-toxins that you can fare as well as the fortunate people who are born and raised all their lives in the Hunza, the Caucausus, the Ecuador and other health Shangri-las. Here is how to use Triple Tonic Secret to minimize, almost to extinction, the effects on your body of added food toxins.

Your Indispensable Trimness Activator

A most important requirement for attaining a healthy, trim, youthful body and a small waist is a sharp thinking mind. You can always possess such a mind because science, without further question, has recently discovered that intelligence does not necessarily decline with age.[6] Dr. Schale's work was lauded by Dr. Jack Botwinick, director of the Aging and Development Program at Washington University in St. Louis, Mo., as one of the most systematic investigations of psychological human development and the effects of aging ever attempted. Dr. Schale said[7] that some persons sink mentally in their 30's, but others "practically never" do so. Some of the best ways to avoid senility, he explained, "include eating well."

Elderly people, he added, were not as likely to grow senile today, because they had more education, better nutrition and health care. Their early life experiences were also more favorable, and they had a "relative absence" of infectious diseases in their childhood.

Dr. Schale had conducted his experiment with 2500 people over a 20-year period. I heartily agree with his conclusions. But I myself was favored by none of these favorable experiences during my early life. Still, I continue making one miracle discovery after another and writing one book after another that is far ahead of my time. While dwelling in the disease-ridden tropics from birth up to my seventeenth year, I caught nearly every infectious childhood disease, except smallpox. Months before coming to the United States I was hospitalized repeatedly with malaria. Except for brief periods in between, I did not conquer all my ills permanently until the age of 30. Yet, today, decades later, I am at my prime mentally and physically. How, you ask, did I achieve it contrary to all of Dr. Schale's 20-year findings?

Eating well is a significant 50 percent of the answer. Not just eating well, but wise eating in combination with *Yogatronics.* With it, I attained a healthy, trim youthful body and a small waist. With it, I counteracted the drastic effects of year-after-year of malnutrition and of poisoned, depleted, big city food. With it, I not only evaded senility, but *increased* my creativity. With it, I even retain my ideal weight for longevity. So can you.

Learn the Triple Tonic Secret to ward off the effects of food poisons. Illustration 12.

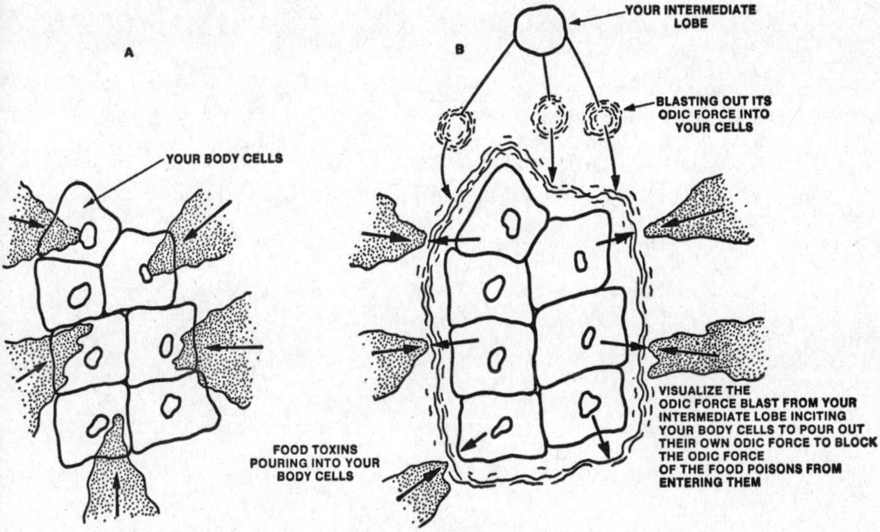

Illustration 12

How Jane C. Greatly Improved Every Phase of Her Life

Jane C. reached a stage, over a period of time, when practically everything she did went wrong. She grew frustrated, ate more, gained weight and went to her doctor for help. He diagnosed her as being in sound health. After watching her eat I concluded that she consumed too much food with sprays and food additives and was saturating her system with poisons which did not affect her clinically, as yet.

I had Jane add the four *Yogatronic Diet* secrets to her diet to ward off the effects of food poisons. These are the very secrets which have apparently preserved me from such toxins after consuming then nearly all my life. Then, she added the Triple Tonic Secret to it.

It wasn't long before Jane was acting like a cat awakening from a long sleep. Her thinking, her daily behavior, her attitudes, her whole demeanor changed—and she lost 23 pounds. She still continued eating poison-saturated, depleted, long-stored supermarket food. I advised her, though, to buy all the organic food she could afford. It was the best food sold to eat—if she could afford it.

REFERENCES

[1]*National Enquirer*, January 31, 1978.

[2]Conducted by Dr. William Bruce, professor of medical biophysics.

[3]Margaret Morrison. March 1975, U.S. Department of Health, Education and Welfare, Public Health Service, Food and Drug Administration Office of Publication Affairs, Publication No. (FDA) 75-2015.

[4]*Stedman's Medical Dictionary*. Eighteenth Revised Edition. (Williams & Wilkins Company. Baltimore.)

[5]Dr. Robert I. Henkin and a group of endocrinologists at the National Institite of Health in Bethesda.

[6]Dr. K. Werner Schale, Director of the University of Southern California Gerontology Research Institute, top psychologist, on a massive study of 2500 persons over a 20-year period.

[7]*Ibid.*

11

yogatronic diet secrets for releasing money-making power

IMPORTANT DIETARY AID TO MAKE YOU A MONEY-MAKER

It takes mental and physical vitality to make substantial money. You don't make it by just thinking about it. You have to plan, direct and even participate in the enterprise. You have to keep a sharp lookout and an alert mind at every step you take. You have to be ready to alter your strategy, your tactics or even your direction when caught by surprise or when your plans don't materialize as you planned. To achieve this most effectively, you have to be in peak health. That is, your body has to be trim and your waist small and firm without fasting, taking drugs, weakening yourself or influencing your mind artificially. Your organs have to feel light, your brain clear and your body springy with muscle tone. You have to feel like a jogger or a sprinter, not like a patient in a wheelchair.

One of your most important dietary aids to achieving this state of mind and body in a daily permanent manner is taking the proper amount of vital minerals regularly. That's why in *Yogatronics* I urge the taking of vitamin-mineral pills on a daily basis. I prefer those made from sea-food, because each seafood specie is very rich in one or more specific minerals. Yet, sea-food contains all the other minerals in small quantities. The American Society of Biochemical chemists reported, as far back as 1941, that no possible combination of synthetic vitamins could support the life cycle, whereas, fruits, vegetables and yeasts can. Sea-food is one of these natural foods. By "seafood" I mean seaweed because only small amounts of shellfish should be eaten.

THE NATURAL YOGATRONIC DIET AIDS FOR MONEY-MAKING POWER

My respect for seafood has not diminished. But, since 1961, I have ceased taking concentrated foods except for a food like powdered kelp. I have found that the natural foods I list in the *Yogatronic Diet* apparently supply all the vitamins and minerals my body needs. My followers agree implicitly.

Science agrees that you *can* feel better, look younger and live longer by taking minerals.[1] These traits are of utmost importance for making substantial money. The *Yogatronic Diet* is replete with foods which are the major sources of the most essential minerals, as listed by two expert nutrition scientists.[2] Here is a list of such foods, culled from the foods recommended for the *Yogatronic Diet.*

They include different foods, or go beyond those listed by the scientists. The *Yogatronic Diet* divides them into 6 groups.

Group 1: Your Blood Builders

Iron is necessary to carry life-giving oxygen through your blood to your tissues. Fine sources are raisins, grapes, eggs, meats, fish, liver, beans, fresh vegetables, whole grain products (which certainly include whole wheat bread and wheat germ) and any whole grain breakfast cereal, like wheat or oats. Nutritionists also include molasses, whole wheat crackers and shredded wheat. I oppose all three additions. All through *Yogatronics* I oppose using sugar, even natural sugar. Sugar is acid, or—through chemical reactions—turns your stomach acid. So it kills your appetite fast. Sweets also create mucus. Not natural sweets, like grapes, but all foods sweetened with any concentrated sweetener, such as sugar or honey. Yes, even honey.

Science upholds me with a most important reason for not eating sugar, not only refined sugar, but even honey or raisins. It found that natural sugar was just as injurious to the teeth and caused just as much tooth decay as refined sugar. Molasses being an exceptionally sticky food, it will obviously fasten even more tenaciously to your teeth and in the crevices of their biting surfaces, causing still more decay. The decalcification (calcium-robbing) potential of figs was the highest measured, and molasses must rank close to them. I myself still eat raisins and figs every day, but I wash my teeth immediately after the meal. I also oppose crackers of any kind because their brittleness wears down your teeth during chewing. So does shredded wheat. The *Yogatronics Diet* recommends seaweed besides those foods recommended by nutritionists, as a very high source of iron, while the nutritionists do not.

Without enough *Copper*, you become anemic. Rich sources are beans, nuts, liver, kidney, brain, seaweed, raisins, grapes, and fresh non-leafy vegetables, like potatoes and carrots. The nutritionists add heart, molasses and bone meal. None of their additions are even listed in the Heinz Table of Dietary Sources of Copper. Yet, the *Yogatronic Diet*, in its regular fare, includes additional very high sources like avocado, oats, wheat, and seaweed (one of the highest sources of copper).

Group 2: Your Organ Builders

Zinc is good for your hair growth, your pancreas and to metabolize your sugar in an emergency. Excellent sources are fish, liver, kidney, brain, shellfish (shrimps, crabs, oysters, scallops), whole grain products and oily nuts. The nutritionists list all of these, but add brewer's yeast, soybeans and spinach. But these foods contain infinitessimal amounts of zinc. Brewer's yeast contains 80 parts per million of zinc; soybeans are not even mentioned in the zinc tables and spinach contains a mere 3-9 parts per million. I, on the other hand, also recommend fish highly as a regular food, for it contains from 700-1200 parts per million of zinc.

Manganese revitalizes your pancreas, kidneys, sex organs, skin, muscle and bones. Liberal sources are bananas, celery, eggs, fresh leafy vegetables, beans, whole grain products and nuts. The nutritionists list all these, but add bran and tea to them. *Yoga-*

tronics cautions about bran. *All-bran* cereals can be 'too rough' for the system. Tea is too acid-creating. Avoid tea, as it is not food and acidifies your system. It is also hard on the kidneys. People who take it as a tonic or stimulant are not feeding themselves with live food. The stimulating effect they bring is only temporary. The stimulating effect which live food brings you, on the other hand, is a natural part of you. It stays with you night and day and even during sleep. You are *more alive* from eating them. When the effects of tea wear off, however, you are *less alive* from consuming it, because your system is *more poisoned* than it was before.

Group 3: Your Muscle Builders

Potassium creates powerful muscle tone and strengthens your nerves. Generous sources are whole grain products, meats, fresh fruits and fresh vegetables, which the nutritionists list. The *Yogatronic Diet*, in addition, includes seaweed, the high source which science apparently omitted or did not mention in the report.

Calcium contributes to your muscle tone, blood-clotting, acid-base balance and a normal heart beat. Liberal sources are dairy products, like skim milk and cheese, and liver, eggs and nuts. The nutritionists list these, but replace skim milk with milk, and add yogurt, bone meal and almonds. I obviously accept almonds, but I still favor skim milk over milk for calcium. It has 199 (per unit measurement), while milk has only 118, and yogurt has 120. In a previous chapter I analyzed bone meal as a food not truly meant for human consumption.

Note: For 24 years, in my books and courses, I repeatedly warned my readers against eating all-bran cereals because they were "too rough" for the system. On Radio CBS 78, January 9, 1978, 24 years later, it was announced that scientists in a leading university, experimenting on rats, have found that bran exposed the intestinal cells to much worse than that. My readers and followers were favored with this knowledge 24 years before it was proved on rats in the laboratory.

Group 4: Your Body and Sex Energy Intensifiers

Chromium eases your body's use of the sugar you consume for energy. Good sources are whole grain products, wheat germ and seaweed. The nutritionists list these and add brewer's yeast, clams and dark brown sugar. But these foods' contents of the trace mineral must be infinitessimal because none of them are listed in the tables.

Sodium increases your protein digestion and sex energy. The great source is seaweed. The *Yogatronic Diet* is absolutely against taking salt. A seaweed like kelp abounds with sodium, iodine, iron, copper and magnesium. It also contains trace elements, like barium, boron, chromium, lithium, nickel, silicon, silver, stronthium, titanium, vanadium and zinc. Salt is not a food. It turns your stomach acid and raises your blood pressure. Although the salt content of your blood is only about 18 percent, you better take more seaweed to make up for the amount of salt you need daily. Many other foods contain sodium, many of which are included in the *Yogatronic Diet*. They include cabbage, celery stalks, chicken leg, dandelion greens, eggs, kohlrabi, lamb, lentils, beef liver, mackerel, stream trout and white turnips.

Group 5: Your Important Body Functions

Iodine normalizes your thyroid, your metabolism gland. The incomparable source is seaweed. The nutritionists list it too. But they add iodized salt. I object, I repeat, to all forms of added salt. Nowhere do I encourage adding salt to food. In fact, foods that fail to arouse a feeling of eagerness and jubilation in you—such as, tasteless foods—still nourish you if they are good foods. Most people try to add taste to their food by fancy cooking and seasoning which includes "salting." But that is no solution, for seasoning, spicing and cooking create acidity. Yes, salt creates an acid stomach, as well as raising the blood pressure.

Phosphorus is necessary for at least 14 of your vital body functions including normal metabolism of muscle, carbohydrate, fat, protein, brain and nerve, blood chemistry, skeletal growth, acid-base regulation, vitamin and enzyme activity. The usual sources are meat, fish, fowl, whole grain products, eggs, cheese and fresh leafy vegetables. The nutritionists also listed these, but add colas and brewer's yeast. I cannot accept their additions. From as far back as *Solar Diet* I never recommended soft drinks, which certainly includes colas. Colas are acid, contain caffeine and erode the teeth. I am surprised that the nutritionists mention these drinks when they contain no food value. These drinks contain only empty calories, which produce quick energy—and fat. The caffeine in them increases the secretion of hydrochloric acid in your stomach, and colas are the most acid of soft drinks.[3] That's why they erode the teeth. Brewer's yeast contains a tremendous amount of phosphorus, but the proportion is 9 times greater than its calcium, which is why I do not recommend brewer's yeast as a safe source of phosphorus.

Group 6: Your Efficient Metabolism

Magnesium is needed for the efficient joining up of the amino acids in you to create proteins. The abundant sources are whole grain products, fresh green vegetables, potatoes and nuts. The nutritionists recommend this identical list, but they add bran and brewer's yeast to it. *Yogatronics* has cautioned you against the excess roughage effect of bran. As for brewer's yeast, it is not even mentioned in the magnesium tables, while oatmeal, which is listed in the tables as another good source of magnesium, is found in the *Yogatronic Diet*.

Selenium is required to protect your liver, for normal metabolism of your red blood cells. The best sources are eggs, beef, fish and beans. The nutritionists announce these, but they add oysters, which are left out of the *Yogatronic Diet* because of the poisons being discovered in oyster beds. These have increased over the years. The best way to get needed minerals, the nutritionists add, is to eat a variable, wide range diet of *un*processed foods, which is exactly what *Yogatronics* consists of.[4] Another prominent researcher, Dr. Emanuel Cheraskin, declares that the best way to get the minerals you need is to eat *un*processed food with mineral supplements, which are usually available only in vitamin-mineral supplements. But, as I have mentioned repeatedly in this book, for the last 15-plus years I have been taking only kelp as a natural supplement.

Dr. Raymond Shamburger, staff biochemist in the clinic biochemistry department at the University of Missouri at Columbia, recently reported that his research team found that heart disease may be related to an insufficiency of selenium in the diet of some victims. Selenium, the article added, is present in seafoods, wheat and rice cereals, garlic and some meats.

IN CONCLUSION

Follow this listing of minerals closely, the leading nutritionists assert today, and you will get the minerals your body needs to "look younger and last longer." You will reclaim your youth and release the vitality you need for money-making powers. With the Triple Tonic Secret (page 49) intensify the amount of minerals you absorb from any food and meet your own varying individual needs.

How Andrew S. Ate Self-Control "Into Himself" and Picked Out Sagacious Ventures to Develop

Andrew S. was shrewd and intelligent. Too frequently, however, he fell under the influence of unresponsiveness. Since he was clinically diagnosed as normal, although he was 30 pounds overweight, I sensed at sight that his organs did not feel light enough to him, that his brain was not as intuitively clear as it could be, and that his body was not springy with muscle tone. He did not feel the clearheadedness of a jogger or a sprinter, but rather seemed like a patient in a wheelchair.

I urged Andrew to eat more mineral-containing foods, and to apply Triple Tonic Secret. In a month, he gained unbelievable control over himself as his weight melted off. He was picking out sagacious ventures to develop, which made him huge profits.

How Marcella M. Sweetened her Moods and Changed Her Husband into an Overwhelming Success

Marcella M. was naturally impatient and had grown worse with her husband's repeated business failures. Ed (her husband) had quit his job to "strike out on his own," and Marcella had contributed her hard-earned savings to help him. But her savings were vanishing alarmingly. Soon, Marcella might have no money left except her Social Security, when she was old enough to collect it. She had gained 41 pounds in weight.

I urged her to eat more mineral-containing foods along with the *Yogatronic Diet*. Within five short weeks she lost nearly 20 pounds, her attitude altered altogether and she became more philosophical and conciliatory towards Ed. His protective tension lessened and he confided his real business problems to her. They worked things out together, and Ed secured another business loan to help him out. The business thrived, and before the end of the year, Ed had converted it into an overwhelming success.

REFERENCES

[1]*National Enquirer*, Nov. 29, 1977. Dr. Emanuel Cheraskin, chairman of the department of oral medicine, University of Alabama, and author of *Psychodietetics*. Dr. Richard Brennan, author of *Nutri-genetics*, and founder of the 500-member International Academy of Preventive Medicine, based in Houston, Tex. Dr. Donald Oberieas, chairman of the department of nutrition and food science at the University of Kentucky. Dr. William Strain, director of the Trace Elements Laboratory at Case Western Reserve University, School of Medicine in Cleveland. Dr. Klaus Schwarz, chief of the Laboratory of Experimental Metabolic Disease, Veterans Administration Hospital, Long Beach, Calif. Dr. Roger J. Williams, University of Texas chemistry professor emeritus and past president of the American Chemical Society.

[2]Dr. Donald Oberieas, a nutritional biochemist with the department of nutrition and food sciences, University of Kentucky. And Dr. Donald R. Davis, a nutrition researcher at the Clayton Foundation Biochemical Institute at the University of Texas.

[3]*Consumer Reports*, July, 1959, following a thorough investigation.

[4]Dr. J. Michael Labe, director of nutrition activity at the U.S. Government's Center for Disease Control in Atlanta.

12

The Yogatronic Secret for a Sharp Thinking Mind

HOW KEEPING YOUR MIND SHARP HELPS YOUR BODY AND WAIST STAY TRIM

Unless you keep your mind sharp, particularly as you get older, it slows down and your body turns fat. Even if you weigh less, the tissues of your "older" body increase in fatty degeneration. To keep your body trim and youthful, you have to live daily with a young mind. You have to be bursting with enthusiasm about something that means a considerable amount to you and over which you have marked control. Your mind has to feel daring and eager to meet new challenges. Once you fall victim to boredom, your mind loses the energy to be active and you put on weight and get a bigger waist.

For nearly thirty years I propounded in my books and courses that you do *not* grow old, either mentally or physically, due to the socalled "aging process," but *only* if you let yourself grow old. By keeping your mind active, flexible and continually growing, I insisted, you prevented it from stagnating and degenerating. I taught, in other words, that senility was far from inevitable.

Nearly three decades later, science upholds me. Marian Diamond, professor of Anatomy in the University of California at Berkeley, conducted experiments on rats whose cells are very much like those of human beings, to test the assertion that you lose up to 100,000 brain cells a day after 30. "No way," she concluded in *Psychology Today.* She failed to find that normal aging (barring the effects of diseases, like hardening of the arteries of the brain) caused brain cell loss, particularly if the subject lived in a stimulating environment. But even when the tests are conducted at various crucial stages of the lives of the subjects, the brain cell loss is trivial.

THE SECRET OF KEEPING YOUR MIND ALWAYS YOUNG

Your brain is unusually active metabolically. Although it weighs approximately only two percent of your total body weight, when you think intensely, its oxygen consumption may rise to as high as 20 or 25 percent of your body's total activitiy. Your brain's metabolism, in other words, is at least *ten times* as active as that of your average tissue (including that of your bones). It has to maintain this high metabolic rate as long as your normal thinking persists. In senility, the total metabolism of the brain is substantially reduced. Under certain anesthetics, like ether and pentathol, brain metabolism may be reduced 30 or 40 percent. The same occurs in diabetic coma.

Since your brain weighs but 2 percent of your total body weight, its efficient use of energy hardly affects the total of your daily need for it. Even the effort involved in solving mathematical problems increases your total metabolism by only 3 or 4 percent. Its fantastic use of energy, though, affects decisively your daily drive to be active, to act wisely and to perform the one exercise in this book which is indispensable to add firmness and more permanency to your waist. It also keeps your telling taste-crave keen and selective instead of being satisfied with food just because of its immediate taste. With my mind constantly hungering to leap far ahead of my time, and popping with miracle discoveries, I have never allowed my mind to stagnate for long. That fact has importantly controlled my weight and kept it "ideal."

HOW NOT TO TRY TO FEED YOUR BRAIN

So-called "brain foods," like fish, are not the primary requisites for your brain to function at its keenest. More important is the avoidance of acidosis, constipation, overeating or overdrinking even of healthy foods or liquids and to limiting your digestion to three square meals a day. Snacks are the enemies of your brain. They draw the blood repeatedly from your brain to your alimentary canal. Certain foods, like apples, mashed potatoes, heavy foods, too much bread, fatty foods (like coconuts, brazil nuts and pecans), whole milk with its fat, roasted nuts, fried foods, big steaks, cheeses, chocolate, cocoa and other foods that digest slowly or with difficulty, cause you to feel sluggish and sleepy. When confronted with complex problems your mind flees then into sexual fantasy and you drowse.

HOW TO FEED YOUR BRAIN WITH THE YOGATRONIC DIET

In contrast, with an alkaline system and with your bowels empty and your waist feeling light, you relish mental challenges and tackle them with vim and vitality and outpace your rivals. The three acid-alkaline balanced square meals of *Yogatronics*, with their two big salads a day, their several servings of fruits and their abstinence from sugar or liquor, is the ideal "wise eating" for mind-sharpening. *Yogatronics* prevents sluggishness by keeping your stomach as empty as possible between meals and allowing your brain to absorb all the nutriment it can from your food.

Mystics and Yogis release the full powers of their minds, but they do so by long fasting and permitting their brains to be freely supplied with blood. Such procedures are impractical in our industrialized society. They also hollow your face and accentuate your years. Besides, no mystics or Yogis are creating books that are far ahead of their time like I am, or making miracle discoveries that take a back seat to nobody—not even to Leonardo de Vinci. So, you don't need to go to the extremes of such wholly dedicated men. Just add the Triple Tonic Secret to the *Yogatronic Diet* and your mind will work at its sharpest. It will also insure your maintenance of a trim body and a small waist—and your ideal weight.

HOW TO MAINTAIN YOUR DAILY EFFICIENCY

"Boring Jobs Actually Make Employees Sick." This represented the newspaper headline of a report by a team of University of Michigan researchers who studied 2,115 American workers in 23 occupations. But, even if you were not bored with your job, or were not under stress from heavy work loads or from carrying much responsibility, you are still likely to get sick *from* it, or *of* it, if your body is not trim, and your waist is not small and hard. When your waist spreads in a formless, unflattering bulk, your whole body loses symmetry, even if it is underweight. (As a rule, however, it adds weight). You *have* to maintain a flat, small, firm waist, or you feel like a nobody, like someone bereft of physical appeal, who is respected only because he is "older" or wields some authority. The usual cause of your shapelessness is eating too much refined sugar, and suffering, as a result, from a deficiency of B-vitamins. Refining sugar removes the B-vitamins which occur naturally in it, and compels your alimentary canal to steal them from other parts of your body.

HOW "ENERGY FOODS" ROB YOU OF ENERGY

Your nerves are the first tissues to be affected by the loss of B-vitamins. The direct cause of the deficiency is usually a diet of soft drinks, candy, sodas, pastries, chewing gum, pies, ice cream—and alcohol. Your attempts to regain your lost "drive" with such "energy foods" fill you only with a quick energy which you lose much too swiftly through your liver. You then feel fatigued, nervous, hungry, restless, dizzy and in time harbor maddening migraine and constipation. You overeat, as a result, to rebuild your "lost energy," and lose your trimness and small waist. Your efficiency at work falters, and you feel "old" and "tired" and in need of a "change." Actually, you need a trim body and a small, firm waist, and your indispositions will vanish.

If you are an executive, or a foreman or your own boss and have to show progress or a profit, you will feel unequal to the task. With a trim body and a small, firm waist, you will feel efficient again.

HOW TO AVOID THE EFFECTS OF "AFTERNOON MENTAL IDIOCY"

No matter how sharp your mind may be in the morning, after a good night's rest and a filling *Yogatronic* breakfast, you have to prevent your mind from losing its peak in the afternoon, after lunch. To prevent that, eat a wise lunch. Don't make lunch a heavy meal. Make breakfast and supper heavy, (despite what others advise about supper, as I will explain in a later chapter), but not lunch. Lunch, in the main, should keep you going until supper. It should also restore the alkalinity of your stomach which your heavy breakfast has changed. A heavy, acid lunch daily leaves you sluggish and tends to constipate you.

A light or alkaline lunch, however, is not meant to be a starvation lunch. A bar of chocolate, or a glass of malted milk and a doughnut, are heavy lunches, even if they appear light. A whole, ripe pineapple or a couple of pounds of grapes—consumed at one time—might fill your stomach, but they are "light" lunches. "Light," in this instance, means easy digestibility. Raw pineapple or raw grapes, can digest in one hour. The more you consume of *any* food, of course, the longer it takes that food to digest. Your stomach has a greater load to handle. Malted milk and a doughnut, or a cup of coffee and a piece of pie or cake, are light in weight compared to several pounds of grapes. But they are 'dead' foods and do not break down easily in the stomach. Being refined foods, they also lack bulk and are compressed by your stomach into hard masses, which tend to "lie like lead" in it.

A FINE, FILLING, HEALTHY LUNCH FOOD

Light food, then, is meant to be raw, alkaline, quickly digesting food. A light meal does not mean limiting your appetite, but implies eating your fill of live, alkaline, quickly digesting food. Finish up your lunch, if you like, with a small quantity of a heavier food like a banana or several dates.

Zucchini is another ideal heavier food. Iowa State University announced on October 25, 1977, in the *National Enquirer*, that the vegetable is both low in calories and high in nutrients. One cup of it contains only 30 calories, or one-third as many as a baked potato.

Zucchini also contains as much vitamin C, thiamin (vitamin B_1), iron and niacin as a potato, and four times the amount of riboflavin. The researchers recommend that you eat zucchini raw, in slices or in a tossed green salad. I prefer to grate it, because chewing off portions of solid foods, such as apples, pears, bread, cheese and, of course, of harder foods, like carrots, will push the gums back, traumatize them, inflame them and engorge them with blood. If repeated, like using a harsh toothbrush, you may eventually end up with gingivitis and bleeding gums, or with pyorrhea or a periodontal disease, which can loosen your teeth. I do not recommend potatoes or beans at lunch, because they make you feel sleepy for the rest of the afternoon. Exception: *boiled* potatoes.

THE LUNCH THAT SHARPENS YOUR MIND

Your afternoon is the second half of your active day. Frequently, it is your most demanding half, the half that requires your shrewdest thinking. Your mind should scintillate until the last instant you work, or you won't appraise the problems you encounter keenly enough or act your wisest. Your wits must be sharp or you won't accurately remember the next day what transpired during the previous afternoon and be able to step forth the next morning as a more capable person. Your lunch should leave you with a satisfied stomach which, before long, feels small again (but not hungry) and keeps your body trim and your waist small.

An excellent big, light lunch dish is a plate of a favorite fruit or a fresh salad bowl. In the last several years I have shifted the salad to breakfast. Meat and cheese sandwiches, pie, ice cream and so on should be avoided as a regular lunch. They take too long to digest and leave you feeling torpid all afternoon. The lunch fruit, however, should not consist solely of light watery fruits, like oranges. Lunch has to last until supper. It should consist of a raw, easily digested fruit or vegetables with some bulk. Pears and peaches (apples give *some* people gas because the skins are hard to digest causing the stomach to secrete so much acid to digest them that they turn sour and fill the stomach with gas) are excellent. Any large quantity of locally grown fruit serves well.

For years now, I have discouraged apples for lunch. They may clean the teeth better than a toothbrush, but they sharpen their edges and thin their enamel coverings. Also, the solid flesh of the apples pushes your gums away from your teeth. Apple skin also lacerates your gums when it slices between your teeth. I advise you, instead, to eat your apples at breakfast with your salad. Grate them, to spare the enamel of your teeth and to protect your gums from the scraping, and from the trauma and erosion by the malic acid they contain. Serve them with your salad, like a dressing.

THE MAGIC WORTH OF APPLES—IF EATEN THE RIGHT WAY

When apples are grated you digest the whole of them, not just particles which happen to be tiny enough after chewing, while less finely chewed particles pass through you unchanged and encourage diarrhea. To masticate apples to a digestible pulp requires considerable chewing. If engaged in regularly it will wear down the biting surfaces of your teeth. You may not be aware of it, but when you chew, you don't chew the food alone; you clash the biting surfaces or your opposing teeth against each other. That's why they wear down quickly. Besides, the friction that takes place in long chewing, such as when you eat an apple or a tough beefsteak, produces unusual heat in your mouth which warms up your teeth and your saliva. The unusual heat activates the eroding malic acid of the apple even more, as well as weakening the resistance of your enamel to erosion, either from the acid (as with the apple), or from the friction of chewing (as with the apple and the tough beefsteak). Also, as your jaws tire from the long mastication, you may start swallowing up to one half of the remaining apple unchewed. It bloats you with gas, and you wonder whether you are "allergic" to apples and should avoid them.

How to Prepare Your Apples and Spare Your Teeth and Gums

Grating the apples (or shredding them very fine) can solve this impasse. You will also enjoy them more and derive far more benefit from them, even if they lose some vitamins during and after the process. You also spare your teeth and your gums from the trauma of chewing them, and you reduce the period of the eroding contact of their acid on your teeth. Apples, however, decalcify (rob) your body *far less* than most foods. (So do carrots.) Their skins contain considerable vitamin C. Since peeling them to escape their sprays robs you of their skins, you should, instead, scrub them vigorously with a hard brush and mild soap to get off all the insecticides you can. Buy organically grown apples (all fruits and vegetables, for that matter) if you can get them and can afford them. If you can't afford them (like me), resort to the stiff brush and soap. Considering the numbers of apples I have eaten daily all these decades, brushing them seems to have served me well. In either case, still grate your apples and eat them for breakfast rather than for lunch. Follow these rules and your lunch will save you from the effects of "afternoon mental idiocy" and sharpen your mind.

WHAT TO DRINK AT LUNCH

Complete your lunch with the lunch beverage. You can finish your lunch with a beverage, if you like. If you have consumed a large, light lunch dish of fruit, you might end your lunch with a glass (or more) of juice of the same fruit, or of a fruit which combines with it. Juices, however, are now concentrated with insecticides, particularly since so much of the food used has to be squeezed to make the juice. This prevents me from recommending them highly. Drink no milk at lunch time, because it takes too long to digest. Milk is an alkalizing food, but it is still a mucous-forming protein. Take little water at meal time. Drink it only between meals, Make your meal time your *food* time, not your water drinking time.

HOW TO STAY MENTALLY KEEN BETWEEN LUNCH AND SUPPER

You hit your low in the middle of the afternoon. This is doubly true in warmer climates, for it is then that the weather is hottest. Many tropical countries have made that the siesta hour. Practically all animals rest at that hour. Quickly advancing twilight, however, makes it difficult to do so in temperate countries.

In midafternoon, too, you feel emptiest. That's why you probably take that perilous afternoon snack which fills doctors' offices and the hospitals with stomach trouble patients, and cemeteries with premature graves. Your afternoon snack may be a social snack with the office bunch (if you work) or with a sociable neighbor or caller (if you don't work) or even because you are bored. You then eat pastries and coffee, tea, or cola drinks or some other stimulant.

With your stomach empty by then, your digestive juices secrete in full and fill your stomach with acid. This kills your appetite for supper, as well as making it difficult for you to digest the snack. Even a Coke, a candy bar or a cocktail—anything whatever, except plain water, which you put into your stomach during the interval between lunch and supper, is fatal to the health of your stomach, to the regularity of your bowels and to your general health. And, of course, it will fill you with gas, enlarge your waist and increase your weight.

Of course you feel somewhat hungry in the middle of the afternoon. And your friends do laugh at you if you refuse to join them in the social snack. You can still join them, however, if you drink only plain water. And you *should* drink several glasses of it between lunch and supper.

THE YOGATRONIC DIET FOR PSYCHIC POWER

Apparently, normal brain tissue can, under adverse circumstances, discharge in a disorganized manner and produce a convulsive seizure.[1] It is the state into which mystics seem to fall. So did many of the prophets in the Bible, including Moses, who was known to fall into "seizures." In this state many of them have had their greatest visions. Some scientists have suggested that the state is brought on by an abnormal concentration of acetylcholine (which stimulates the parasympathetics) in the damaged area of the brain which renders them more reactive to stimuli. According to Merck, however, the evidence for that hypothesis is lacking.

I feel that these scientists hit the mark on the head. I myself fell most easily into the state of Zodic Ecstasy super-sensitivity, for instance (which I describe in ZODIC FORCE CONTROL), when I lived on a vegetarian diet or was half-starved from lack of funds to buy food and drank a lot of water to feel full. My body was most alkaline then. In that state my parasympathetic nervous system was predominant in my body. A pathological example of such a condition is in Addison's disease. It is the result of a lessened functioning of the adrenal gland, with a resulting predominance of the parasympathetics over the weakened functioning of the sympathetics. The afflicted person tastes and smells far more keenly than the normal person and hears sounds which the normal person cannot.

Pychologically, he is closest to the psychic receptivity of a mystic.

Potassium, not calcium, rules your parasympathetics. You also need potassium for water balance. Foods with too much sugar or protein (like dates, meat and beans) turn your body acid and bring on a predominance of your sympathetics, which are ruled by calcium, thus reducing your psychic powers.

FOODS TO PUT YOU AT YOUR PSYCHIC BEST

To be at your psychic best for everyday life, don't overeat even naturally concentrated foods, like dates or figs, or even good proteins, like beans or meats. You do need them for muscle repair, to build your cells and to prevent your face and body from looking too lean. But limit the dates you eat to from four to six a day if you are physically active, and the dried figs to three a day. If you tend to gain weight easily, reduce your dates or figs to one or two a day. Follow the *Yogatronic Diet* closely otherwise, especially in respect to eating fruits and vegetables and keeping your acidosis down to a minimum. If you do strenuous exercise, double the dates.

For keenest psychic reception, I would even advise you to wash out your sinuses with very warm salt water once a day, before supper or before going to bed. Fill a container with the warm salt water, bend over low and immerse your nose in the water. Snuff it up into your nostrils and down into your mouth and spit it out. Do this about four times. Then wash the salt water out of the lower nostrils where it might collect, and gargle a little to prevent swallowing any salt water. Blow your nose *gently* several times afterwards to clear it altogether. Not only will this help to keep you free of colds and other respiratory infections, but it will clean your sinuses so thoroughly that you will hear much better, more like a psychic. Every diet, except a strict vegetarian or fruit diet, accumulates a certain amount of mucus in your sinuses every day. This blocking mucus reduces some of your oxygen intake and the keenness of your senses. By cleaning your sinuses daily with salt water, you extract this regularly accumulated mucus. Your head will feel much clearer and you will receive impressions from all around you which you were hardly aware of before. Your voice will gain tremendously in resonance by morning. After all the water has drained your sinuses, add the Triple Tonic Secret (Page 49) to this sinus-cleaning and you will swiftly possess an undreamed of psychic power for everyday life.

How John B. Was Promoted Unexpectedly at Retirement Age

John B. worried more and more as he neared retirement age. Contrary to his employer's opinion, I felt that his mind was sharp enough to compete successfully with his younger rivals. It was merely being clouded by his acidosis-creating diet. John carried 25 extra pounds of "acid weight," as I called it.

With the *Yogatronic Diet*, John ate his fill, as before, but lost weight. His head cleared, as if he had rid himself of the daily catarrh resulting from excess carbohydrate and protein. His waist lost several inches, and he felt youthful and flexible again. In a surprisingly short time, he acted, thought—and looked—like a much younger man. Instead of being retired, he was unexpectedly promoted over younger men to make use of his long job experience.

How Ellen K. Lost 37 Pounds and Out-Thought Her Rivals

Ellen K. worked in a very competitive field that required the utmost tact, keen judgment, a close eye on the changing times and the sensing of future customer desires and needs. A minor mistake of hers could prove costly to her company and cause her dismissal. Her position demanded so much of her that she paid little attention to what she ate, lost her mental sharpness and put on considerable weight.

With the *Yogatronic Diet* Ellen was again blessed with full bowel movements and lowered her acidosis. She lost 25 pounds, and her waist thinned and released her hidden powers. She gained a psychic ability, a special intuition and a sensitivity to recognize the most successful plans to pursue. She intensified it remarkably with the Triple Tonic Secret.

In 12 or 13 weeks she had lost a total of 37 pounds. But her face, to her relief, still looked comparatively full. She out-thought her rivals and made one astoundingly wise decision after another for her company. There was talk of making her its first female vice-president.

REFERENCES

[1]*The Merck Manual of Diagnosis and Therapy.* Merck & Co., Inc., Rahway, N.J., 1956.

13

yogatronics—the magic way to a svelte waistline

THE SINISTER EFFECTS OF ATROPHY

Certainly you can acquire a slim waistline by altering your diet, such as, by fasting or taking special food preparations, and doing no exercise. But this is what will happen to your body, according to Boyd's *Pathology*, page 215.[1] (Italics and squared parentheses insertions are mine).

> Atrophy is a diminution in size, a shrinking of cells or fibers which have reached their full development. . . . Atrophy may occur under a great variety of different conditions. Some of the most important of these are old age, *lack of nourishment*, disuse, the action of toxins, pressure and interference with nerve supply [such as, subluxations of your spine from habitual bad posture]. As *age* advances there is a general tendency towards atrophy, best seen in the uterus, ovary, breast, lymphoid tissue, and bone marrow. Chronic *starvation* causes wasting of adipose tissue and *muscles;* atrophy also follows decreased blood supply due to *arteriosclerosis*. *Disuse* of a structure results in atrophy. . . .

Boyd, then, states that atrophy may be caused by *old age, lack of nourishment, disuse of a structure, wrong posture, chronic starvation,* and, or by, *hardening of the arteries.* Atrophy, he explains, can occur in the muscles, the organs of the body and the bone marrow. The atrophied organ, in other words, may be visible and is closely linked with the appearance of an organ like the breasts. That's the kind of atrophy which you bring upon yourself when you fast or try to lose weight with special food preparations alone, instead of with wise eating. You age yourself prematurely with them and shrink from head to foot, including the muscles of your face and heart. Your organs shrivel and function less efficiently, reducing your energy, your vitality and your length of life. The covering muscles of your body wither and leave you shapeless and less V-shaped. Your waist may be smaller, but only because your abdominal muscles and your viscera are emaciated.

HOW FASTING ACTUALLY FATTENS YOU WHILE YOU FAST

Fasting, besides, significantly suppresses your sympathetic nervous system, your nervous survival system of "fight or flight," of energy and activity, of combatting disease, of the drive to compete and win in any field, of mental alertness. This occurs in the heart, liver, pancreas, spleen, small intestine and salivary glands, indeed, in all the organs examined, and appears to "reflect changes throughout the organism."[2] The reason given is that your body suppresses your sympathetics when you fast, to try to save calories. So—the researchers suggest that "manipulation to increase" the activity of the sympathetics may be important for treating obesity. To state it briefly, when you fast, your body tries to save calories and *makes you fatter* to help you survive the lack of food. Simultaneously, since you are inactive, your body atrophies (that is, your muscles, your organs, your bone marrow, etc.), and you get thinner *but smaller all over, even in the places you don't want to shrink.*

HOW TO GET BIGGER AND SMALLER IN THE RIGHT PLACES—WHILE GETTING THINNER

When you are active or exercise systematically, your body throws off calories and you also get thinner. Your muscles and your organs *build up,* however, and you get *bigger and smaller in the right places.* To fast or lose weight through inactivity (unless under the orders of your professional healer) amounts to doing to your body what old age does to it: that is, *to atrophy* it. But, your goal is to be trim and possess a small waist, not to look old and feeble. *That's* what the *Yogatronic Diet* does for you. By permitting you to eat your fill, it retains your desirable filled-out parts and keeps you looking young as long as possible. With its twice-a-day fibrous salad, however, it decreases your fat-intake and controls your weight. With the Abdominal Double Curl you contract your waist and make it firm. With the Triple Tonic Secret you absorb the most nutriment from your food. You look younger and trimmer as a result. You are also much stronger and healthier, because your heart and your organs have not atrophied, but have been built up instead.

SUMMARY OF BOYD'S SIX CAUSES OF ATROPHY

Here, in a nutshell, are Boyd's six causes of atrophy in your body and the consequent loss of your trimness and small waist.

1. Lack of nourishment. [To be more exact, lack of enough nourishment in your food, even if you overeat].
2. The action of toxins. [Such as a diet of junk food, or of a processed, stored-too-long diet saturated with insecticides, dyes, emulsifiers or other additives].
3. The gradual hardening of your arteries [by cholesterol plaques forming around their inner surfaces].
4. Bad posture, [usually from your occupation, which distorts the normal alignment of your vertebrae and disrupts your correct body mechanics].
5. From disuse [such as lack of sufficient muscle toning exercises, as distinguished from fatiguing, wearying or exhausting efforts like housework, gardening, tennis, water-skiing, golf or marathon running].
6. Premature or normal aging.

Any, or all, of these health traumas will deprive you of filled-out body trimness and a small, firm waist. Learn, now, the *Yogatronic Secrets* to avoid each one.

Secret 1. How to Bypass the Youth-Ruining Dangers of Lack of Nourishment when Keeping Trim

You will not atrophy from lack of nourishment or lose your trimness if you eat large meals daily but follow the wise eating of the *Yogatronic Diet*, as revealed throughout this book.

Secret 2. How to Rout the Action of Toxins on Your Youth-Seeking Body

You already learned how in Chapter 10, page 129.

Secret 3. How to Nullify Gradual Hardening of the Arteries and Stay Youthful and Trim

Your arteries harden gradually with age, but they harden faster when cholesterol deposits on their inner surfaces. The resulting plaques prevent your arteries from dilating and constricting as easily and effectively as they did before and reduce the volume of blood which they supply to different parts of your body. The alkaline diet is the fastest one to nullify the gradual hardening of your arteries. To clarify your understanding of an alkaline diet I will now explain the meaning of dietary acidosis and of an over-alkaline diet.

THE TRUE MEANING OF DIETARY ACIDOSIS

Don't confuse the effects of an over-alkaline diet with those of alkalosis resulting from drinking quarts of orange juice at one time. The term "acidosis" was originally introduced by Naunym (1838-1925) to signify the production in your body of the abnormal acid metabolites beta-hydroxybutyric and acetoacetic acids. These acids are "ketone bodies." They are found in excess in severe diabetes, in the "acidosis" of childhood and during anesthesia. They can be triggered by an unbalanced diet containing high fats and carbohydrates.[3] The "ketone bodies" are normal degradation products of the fatty acids and are formed in your liver. Your liver dispatches them into your bloodstream, which distributes them all over your body. Hence, acidosis results from eating foods that add to your weight and coat the inner surfaces of your arteries with cholesterol, turning them prematurely sclerotic. It converts your arteries into fibrous tissue which does not stretch or contract like functioning muscle, and which, for that reason, is commonly called "hardening of the arteries." To avoid "acidosis," the obvious step is to eat food that causes alkalinity, not acidity: to eat foods with the least fat, which fatten you least.

THE DRAWBACKS OF OVER-ALKALINITY

An over-alkaline diet, on the other hand, overstimulates your system and drives you into living at too rapid a pace. It won't shorten your life; indeed, the more alkaline the diet, the longer you are likely to live.

But there is a condition known as "alkalosis." It has been purposely induced by the administration of large quantities of sodium bicarbonate (bicarbonate of soda) for therapeutic reasons, or by the drinking of huge amounts of fruit juice or water at the same time, to the point of causing "water intoxication" and incapacitating abdominal gripes. People have died from eating too many oranges, pears or other fruits at one time. Inspect the inscriptions on many a tombstone in the early 19th century.

But, let's continue with the normal diet which is made over-alkaline by omitting practically all fats. Over-alkalinity trims your weight down to an unflattering degree and leaves you feeling so 'light' that you become restless and overenergetic. Mystics and Yogis go on long fasts or alkalize their systems with non-acid foods—and *train* themselves to harness this excessive energy and use it for their "miraculous" purposes. By shaking off every ounce of fat until you are practically lean flesh and bone, (even atrophying your bone marrow), you add to your power of mind the energy which you would expend otherwise to pump blood through your fat.

From the standpoint of your appearance, however, this total loss of fat is unflattering. It hollows your cheeks, carves circles under your eyes, protrudes your collarbones and ribs, and adds years to your looks. Whether you are a man or a woman, losing your looks is the last thing you want to do. To look young, you have to keep fat on your face and body, but don't keep enough on them to imperil your health.

THE WISE ALKALINE DIET

Here, with my up-to-date comments, is the wise alkaline diet which keeps your blood pressure down and helps prevent the hardening of your arteries, which in turn keeps you active, your waist small and your body trim without starving, fasting, taking food preparations or even vitamins. *The Alkaline Diet:* A fruit or two, like the orange, needs grapefruit or lemon juice added to it to alkalize it more easily in your stomach. Practically all alkaline *fresh* fruit or vegetable diets, then, like the grape cure and others, are equally effective alkalizers of the system. The emphasis is placed on *fresh* fruits because, once a fruit is dried it becomes too sweet—like the raisin—or too acid—like the dried prune, the dried peach, the apricot—to remain truly alkaline. As a rule, then, practically *any* fruit used for a diet, is equally effective as a 'diet cure.' Cranberries, which turn to hippuric acid, which is excreted by the kidneys, are one exception. I would avoid them, unless under professional treatment for your kidneys, because they erode the teeth. It requires too much added sugar to reduce their acidity, and that would remove their benefits.

STILL EAT MEAT FOR AN ALKALINE DIET

In brief, still eat lean meats, nuts and skim milk to supply your body daily with necessary fat to feed your nerves and skin, and to save yourself from looking prematurely old, from acquiring unflattering hollows and from atrophying organs. When meat is eaten with an alkaline food (like the salads or watermelon) it acts more like an acid. When eaten with another meat—particularly with a still more acid meat—it acts more alkaline. But, eat a preponderance of fruits and vegetables to prevent your better-fed body from developing hardening of the arteries and thereby shortening your life and health. Help your body extract the utmost benefit out of such soil-depleted, sprayed, over-stored and sadly processed food with the Triple Tonic Secret (page 49). Add the Abdominal Double Curl, page 61, to draw in your waistline firmly, to keep your bowels functioning easily, to squeeze the bloating gas out of you, to bolster your diaphragm and your visceral organs higher in your abdominal cavity and to reward you with a healthy and svelte waist that attracts the eye.

How Louisa G. Altered her Image and Was Soon Eagerly Pursued.

Louisa G. was distraught with her lonely life. Even at work, others practically ignored her. Her figure apparently excited no one, and her waistline contrasted too little with her shoulders or hips. It was obvious to me that the atrophy of disuse and the lack of an alkalizing diet had closed her path to happiness. She was about 60 pounds overweight.

With the *Yogatronic Diet* and the Abdominal Double Curl, Louisia's waistline assumed a svelte look with stunning speed. Her image changed strikingly from day-to-day. Her abdomen drew in firmly as her wasting abdominal muscles sprang back to life. Her breasts, in contrast, seemed larger. People who had ignored her before, paid close attention to her now, and her defeated attitude disappeared. In no time, she was avidly pursued by others, which altered her whole life.

How Richard P. Suddenly Resembled a Successful Actor Rather than an Overworked Father of Four

Richard P. resented looking like an overworked father of four. His family didn't mind, but *he* did. He felt that he should always look fit. In his career, he competed with less-pressed rivals who did not look like overworked parents and he was tired of taking a back seat to them. His clothes got tighter, and he gained 42 pounds on the scale.

Richard convinced his wife that he wanted to eat the *Yogatronic Diet*. His whole family, to his delight, enjoyed it and felt much better from it. Richard was thrilled as his clothes grew loose again, and the weight on the scale dropped. He seemed taller again, his shoulders appeared broader, and he felt much lighter. Aided by the Triple Tonic Secret, this new image of himself was implanted all over him and people took him for being much younger than he was. In seven weeks, he lost 30 pounds and resembled a successful actor more than an overworked father of four.

REFERENCES

[1]William Boyd, M.D., D.Sci. *A Text-book of Pathology: An Introduction to Medicine. Sixth Edition. (Lea & Febiger, Philadelphia p. 215. Reprinted with permission of the publisher).*

[2]J.B. Young and L. Landberg, "Suppression of Sympathetic Nervous System During Fasting," *Science* Vol. 196, No. 4297, pp. 1473-1475, 24 June 1977. American Association for the Advancement of Science, © 1977. Quoted by special permission from *Science* and the authors.

[3]*Human Biochemistry.* Israel S. Kleiner, Ph.D. Fourth Edition, 1954. The C. V. Mosby Co., St. Louis.

14

yogatronics – the magic way to a svelte waistline cont'd

Secret 4. Unnecessary Energy Sapping that Intensifies Your Body's Daily Needs for Calorie-Energy

Aside from an uncontrolled appetite, the main threat to your acquiring and maintaining a trim body and a svelte waistline is your body's steady call for excess energy-calories to help it perform its daily activities without falling victim to fatigue, to lessened efficiency, to loss of motivation, to pessimism, to acceptance of defeat, to antisociality, to anger at monotony, to the tension of decision-making and to the despair of unavoidable problems to face. Your body regularly calls for excess calories, because you waste too many by not conserving them when you easily can. When you keep standing, for instance, when you could easily sit down, you waste an extraordinary amount of body energy resisting the pull of gravity with the anti-gravity muscles of your feet, legs, abdomen, back, shoulders, chest and neck. You waste even more when you sit for long on a poorly designed chair without enough space for your hips to spread, and with no arms for your forearms to rest on. You have to sit unnecessarily straight instead and overwork your back muscles to the point of fatigue trying to maintain that posture, or let yourself slump forwards or sidewards and curve your spine abnormally and compress the important big nerves that supply your organs and your blood vessels, including your heart.

Or you are confined to a swivel-chair on which you lean back, but which also confines your hips from relieving your spine of much of the weight of your back. The seat is perhaps too long and obstructs the circulation near your knees. The movement of the swivel shifts the center of gravity up and down your spine and exhausts its big and small muscles. At home, you slump backwards in an ill-designed armchair and cram your torso on the base of your back. Your body exhausts itself combatting such strains all day, and you have little energy left to draw in your waistline or to care whether you eat wisely or not.

The magic chair that can reduce daily your body's needs for excess calorie-energy

A simple way to conserve a lot of your energy during work (if you can manage it) and certainly at home (where you can manage it) is to sit in a straight-backed chair with arm rests. (Illus. 13B1). Its back should not be high, but high enough to support your lower back. (See Illus. 13B2). The back of the chair should be open below to let your hips slide backwards enough to maintain the natural curve of your back. (See Illus. 13B3). Rest your forearms on the arms of the chair, (See Illus. 13 A 4 & C 4) and lean forward enough to bring the weight of your torso off your back muscles and let your resting forearms support it. (See Illus. 13 A 5 & C 5). You won't look like a straining fashion-model, but you won't look ungraceful either, because your shoulders will appear much broader (if you are a man). If you are a woman, the groove between your breasts will look much deeper. Your back will hardly tire all day, and your spinal discs will not be compressed continuously by gravity. (They are compressed by it when you sit straight, and they wear out and shorten your height decades before your time. Also sit in such a chair at home. Let it conserve your energy for hours every night before going to bed, as well as on weekends, when you read or study or sit to relax.

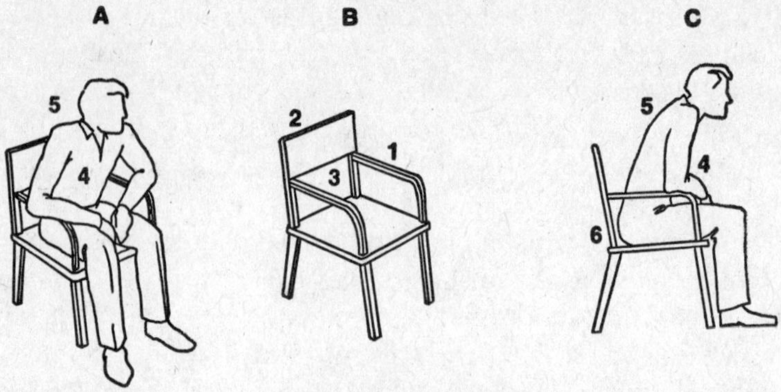

Illustration 13

If you cannot dictate the kind of chair you wish to sit on at work, rest whenever you can by sitting with your forearms resting on your thighs, pointing inwards about 60 degrees, with your hands almost meeting. (See Illus. 13 A). In the magic chair, however, always sit with your pelvis fully back in it. (Illus. 13 C6). Don't sit with your hips placed farther forwards than your back, as the swivel-chair, the back-ruining reclining chair, and most decorative chairs compel you to do. Such chairs compel you to throw your weight upon the delicate base of your spine and the weaker joints of your vertebrae instead of upon the big hip bones of your pelvis to leave your spine relaxed and freed of the load.

Secret 5. One Special Yogametric Exercise to Discourage Unwanted Tissue Atrophy

(The Abdominal Double Curl. Page 61).

Secret 6. How to Retard Your "Getting Old" to the Maximum

Aging is the catastrophic culmination of a group of bad habits in which you persist over most of your life. They include bad habits in nutrition, of dress, of overconcern with pleasure, in recreation, in occupation, and in exercise—in practically everything you do. Alter them and you can double, triple or even quadruple your lifespan. You can continue living to 300 or 400, or "indefinitely," as I affirmed to Jeff Lyon in my long interview with him for his column "Close Up," in the *Chicago Sunday Tribune,* August 14, 1977. *One week* later, leading Russian scientists announced that they were finding that the lifespan of man should reach 400. (I beat them to the punch again). The Russians performed this experiment by injecting placental fluid or other hormones into rats and dogs.

I insist you *can* do it, however, *without* such substances being injected into your body and without your risking their side effects. Age *can* be reversed (or delayed "indefinitely") with diet—with the *Yogatronic Diet.* I myself am doing it, and my scores of miracle discoveries have been repeatedly ahead of science for from 1 to 57 years.

A few decades back, Dr. Alexis Carrel proved that the toxin-drained test-tube organ did *not* die of old age. *You* don't have to, *either.* You, too, can drain the toxins out of yourself and limit the amount of new toxin you take in. You can do so, primarily, by controlling the volume of mucous in you with mucous-destroying food. Beans are a good substitute for meat in your supper, but they are inclined to fill you with mucous and gas. Corn should be eaten fresh, when its kernels are still tender. When cooked, its skins turn thick and indigestible and cannot be chewed fine enough. When swallowed, this covering fills you with gas and passes through you undigested. On the nights when you eat a strong mucous-forming food like cooked potato, double up on your serving of garlic or garlic pills to help neutralize it. *Note:* I always recommend any fresh food in place of its pill form.

My answer to the study that eating fried foods lengthens life

From the 3-year survey of 422,000 men (Hammond Report of 1963), Yale professor Dr. Harold Morowitz recently pointed out that it distinctly showed that men who ate fried food lived longer than those who didn't. The deaths among men who ate *no* fried food was *72% higher* than among those who ate fried foods more than 15 times a week. In fact, the report found, the more fried food the men ate, the longer they lived. I don't believe that this proves the value of fried food. Fried foods, however, do take much longer to digest, and that encourages one not to snack. The report, then, unsuspectingly proves that *snacks* between meals *shorten the length of life.*

The part of your meal that makes you prematurely old

Dessert is the most dangerous food of any meal, as it is difficult to choose one that will not wreck your health. It has to be delicious or you won't enjoy it. Most people, in fact, eat their meals with the dessert in mind. It is the big surprise of the meal, the big thing which the housewife has devoted most of her time to prepare. For that reason, it is the most delicious part of the meal—and also the fastest and surest health-ruining part. The dessert is usually the most indigestible part of your meal, the one that lies longest in your stomach, the most fattening one and the one which, when overindulged, can lead most quickly to trouble. Yet, hardly a soul enjoys his supper without a dessert to look forward to at the end of it.

The usual dessert is a health ruiner. As a rule, it contains white sugar and degerminated white flour, is constipating and mucous-forming and is so thoroughly baked or otherwise altered in its natural composition that it has lost most of its vitamins and other "live food" qualities. If it contains any fruit, the fruit has been sugared and cooked until it is only fruit in name. Its parts have been cut into small bits and exposed to air for so long that they are vastly altered as food. The numerous flavorings and seasonings added to it have not helped it nutritionally. Its overdelicious taste oversecretes saliva which goes into your stomach and leads to acidosis. Being more or less indigestible, it lies in your stomach for hours, hardens into "concrete" in your intestines and all but drags out your rectum with it at the stool. It fills your system with calcium-absorbing white sugar, which robs your teeth and bones of calcium and of vitamin B, which your body needs to digest it, and hardens your arteries comparatively early. Pies, cakes and sweets of all kinds—even ice cream, if regularly consumed—fill your system with acid and mucous and are hard to digest. And, of course, they fatten your figure and enlarge your waistline. When you eat ice cream, avoid soda fountain concoctions, like sodas, malted milks and sundaes. You can get away with a little dissipation now and then, but never dissipate to the point where it takes you time to recover. Your youth lasts longest when you dissipate the least. Have your fun, but don't keep irregular hours and abuse your stomach.

How to eat desserts but stay young

Don't live so soberly that life turns grim and depressing. Live a healthy life *naturally*. You don't have to get drunk and dissipate to enjoy yourself. Indeed, you can enjoy yourself most when you keep your wits wide awake and thrill others with your sparkle and humor.

So, you don't have to deny yourself all enjoyable desserts. Eat those that taste delicious, but that don't hurt you. A dish of stewed prunes not only tastes delicious but also adds to your vitality and eases the passage of waste through your intestines. I wouldn't recommend eating this frequently, because prunes contain a large amount of oxalic acid. Also, the wrinkles on their dried skins are filled with sprays. A slice of avocado is also a tasty and healthy dessert. Too big a slice, however, fattens.

How to Select Mucus-Removing Foods

To repeat, fresh pineapple, apples, watermelon, citrus fruits and tomatoes are excellent mucus-killing foods, and should be made a steady part of your diet. . . . The fresh food available in most stores, of course, is *not* the fresh food eaten from the tree or the ground. And yet, today, I am in perfect health and have lived on such second choice food all my life. But fresh food from city stores can still grow when planted, unless seriously withered.

Eat little of foods which, when cooked, cause mucus. Grate or shred hard vegetables like parsnips, carrots and beets, and eat them fresh. Squash (winter variety) may be baked. It is better, however, to grate the food raw and eat it. Grind, grate or shred fresh pineapple. It's delicious. Potatoes, when grated and eaten raw, *do not fill* you with mucus, and fatten you *much* less than if baked. In fact, they fatten you much less than believed, unless fried or buttered or cooked in some way with fat. But, you might not enjoy their peculiar taste when raw. Boil them, in that event, until they are just soft enough to be pierced one-third through with a sharp fork. Don't cook them until they are too soft, or they lose much of their vitamin C. To save their boiled water is not enough to save many of their vitamins. Don't chew the potatoes when they are still hard. Like apples, they sharpen your teeth, thin down their enamel, push back your gums to the roots of your teeth and inflame them and turn your teeth supersensitive. When cooked, the potato skin turns thick and indigestible and cannot be chewed fine. After you swallow it, it fills you with gas and passes through you undigested. As I explained earlier, the food that is hard to the touch (like raw beets and carrots) is *not* necessarily the hardest food to digest. In fact, once grated or shredded fine, such a food is usually the easiest to digest and excrete because of its natural bulk. Its natural bulk also makes it an ideal mucus-removing food.

Other Ways to Select Mucus-Killing Foods

Beans are a good substitute for meat, but they are inclined to fill you with mucous and gas. It is better to eat raw peas. They are filled with natural energy and *will not* fill you with gas and mucous. The same is true of all cooked fruits and vegetables. When eaten raw and bolted, of course, they do blow you up with gas and stretch the girth of your waist for hours. Apples and other fruits with coarse skins take long to digest because of their thick hard skins. Always grate or shred such fruits before eating them. Even grapes with thick skins fill people with gas. Fruit skin is like the leather taken off an animal. When the fruit is dried, like the raisin and the prune, the skin is still harder to digest. That's why prunes and raisins should be tenderized somewhat before being eaten. If you suffer from stomach trouble, avoid fruits with thick leathery skins or with skins that cannot be grated down fine before putting into the mouth. Leathery skins cause your stomach to secrete so much acid to digest them that it turns your stomach sour and fills you with gas.

Because pasteurized milk is a partly dead food, has lost much of its natural vitamins and contains much butterfat, it may form mucus in many, particularly in those who exercise little. Milk, nevertheless, is a valuable food and cannot be left out of your diet. I assert this despite science's claim that there are people who lack a necessary enzyme in the stomach to digest the galactose in milk. I insist that these people engage in too much activity after eating milk. Garlic being a potent blood cleanser, will markedly lessen the amount of mucus any food forms in your body. So, don't stop drinking milk because of the possibility of your developing mucus. Mucus is not desirable, of course, because it is a fertile ground for germs to grow in. But garlic will help neutralize most of it and fight off germs besides.

A COMPREHENSIVE YOGATRONIC DIET LIST OF ACID-FORMING (MUCUS-FORMING) AND ALKALI FORMING (MUCUS-KILLING) FOODS

Meat, fish and fowl are acid-forming (mucus-forming). Fruits and vegetables are alkali-forming (mucous-killing). That's why you can't tell whether a food is acid or alkali by its taste. Many persons are sensitive to orange juice, tomatoes and similar acid-tasting foods. When they indulge in them they suffer from heart burn, acid conditions and wet burps, because of the excess hydrochloric acid these generate in their gastric juice. The victims call it "allergy."

To be in your best health, however, you should eat slightly more *alkali*-forming over acid-forming foods. But don't eat a markedly predominant amount of either. Scientists have questioned this premise lately, and high protein diets are being urged instead. Nonetheless, the numbers of vegetarians who develop or die from heart disease is still but a minor fraction of that of non-vegetarians, and the vegetarians eat an alkaline diet.

Acid-forming foods consist of meats, fish, fowl, eggs, cereal, pastries and puddings, breads of all kinds (rye, wheat, etc.), oysters. *Alkaline foods* consist of vegetables and fruits. Milk and most nuts are alkaline. Peanuts and cashew nuts are acids, but coconuts are alkaline. Coconuts, though, contain too much saturated fat.

A COMPREHENSIVE YOGATRONIC DIET LIST OF NON-ALKALINE FORMING AND ALKALI FORMING (MUCUS-KILLING) FOODS

Among the non-alkaline forming fruits are: cranberries, plums, prunes, rhubarb. They contain hippuric and other acids which render your urine acidic. Among the *non-alkaline forming vegetables* are: corn, dried lentils. *Neutral foods*, which form neither acid or alkaline, are: various oils (vegetable), butter, cream, lard, sugar (white), corn starch and tapioca. When eaten with pastries and puddings, though, the neutral foods can be acid forming. All the foods in this paragraph are mucus formers, so I don't recommend them, with the exception of prunes. Since you should seek to alkalize your system more often than turn it acid, the following foods are the most efficient alkalizers, in the order named: apples, oranges, bananas, pineapple, potato, muskmelon, carrots, almonds, raisins, dried beans, dried lima beans. They can lower your urinary acidity effectively between 24-48 hours. Water can lower it even faster, but few sources even mention it.

Other alkaline foods are: artichokes, asparagus, beet greens, broccoli, celery, chards, cucumbers, endive, chicory, leeks, lettuce, parsnips, potatoes (white), rhubarb, spinach, squash, summer squash, watercress, apricots, avocados, currants, dried dates, dried figs, gooseberries, guavas, mangoes, nectarines, olives, grandine, peaches, pears, quince, plums, and tangerines.

Certain alkaline foods like spinach and rhubarb contain high amounts of oxalic acid. I have listed them, but don't recommend them as alkaline foods. The vegetarian diet, however, may lack vitamin B_{12} (dobione) because vegetables are practically devoid of them. Good sources of this vitamin are milk, cheese, liver and beef. That is why the *Yogatronic Diet* consists of both acid and alkaline foods. To reduce your calories, if you wish to lose weight, dieticians urge you to substitute a variety of whole grain products for your cereal and bread, and vegetable oils for your butter. True, a research study of late announces that peanut butter, for some enigmatic reason, forms plaques faster or more easily around the inner surfaces of the arteries than any other food. I cannot reply to this conclusion one way or another, but neither can I find a scientific explanation for it. I myself am continuing daily to cover my two thin slices of bread with lean coatings of pure, natural, untampered peanut butter. But I also exercise vigorously five days a week, eat fibrous salads twice a day and two cloves of raw garlic at least three times a week. Further research, I feel, will discover that raw, unroasted, unprocessed peanut butter is a fine and safe food.

To help keep your system alkaline, eat fresh garlic and onions with your meat and potatoes as it tremendously lessens any overacidity that might form. Even eating a good salad with it seems to work. Meat and potatoes, or bread and meat, *might* cause some acidosis if your whole meal was predominently acid. Otherwise, there is no harm in eating meat with potatoes, or meat with bread. If your stomach is acid, tomato juice is excellent for it. So is water and pineapple juice. Fresh garlic and onions actually reduce acidosis for any reason.

The Triple Tonic Secret, which maintains your system more alkaline than acid and leads you on the magic way to a svelte waistline, is on page 71. (Illus. 7).

How Tom and Laura F. Transferred Themselves from the "Sleepy" Group to the "Living" Crowd

Tom and Laura F. had reached the age where they were considered neither young nor old. But since the young generally prefer the younger, they were shunted off into the "sleepy" crowd. Their visions of a lively social life for most of their lives were dissipating into thin air, and they were frightened.

With the *Yogatronic Diet*, Tom and Laura were soon aware that they were regaining the appearance of youth which they had subtly lost. They shed from 20 to 25 pounds apiece, shrank several inches on their waists and acquired vigorous body tones. The "living" crowd eyed them closer wherever they went and accepted them again. Tom and Laura felt as if born again.

How Rudy V. Reduced his Yearly Colds to a Minimum

Rudy V. caught several colds a year, and they lingered on and weakened him. I agree with vegetarians that you catch a cold because your body is acid, for acid is a fertile environment for bacteria. With the *Yogatronic Diet* Rudy lost 28 "acid pounds" faster than he ever dreamed he would. Every night before going to bed, he rinsed his sinuses with warm salt water. He gargled with warm salt water after coming home from work, to sterilize his throat from any microorganisms that might have lodged in it all day long while he had been among other people. With the *Yogatronic Diet* to keep down his acidosis, his head felt very clear again. Year after year, thereafter, Rudy hardly caught a cold. And whenever he did, it lasted very briefly and he did not feel weak from it.

15

yogatronic secrets for restoring the ideal shape of your thighs and calves

HOW IMPORTANT YOUR LEGS ARE TO KEEP YOUR BODY TRIM AND YOUR WAIST SMALL

You cannot expect to gain a firm, small waist and a trim, toned-up body unless your thighs and calves are toned up, too. As I stated repeatedly, a flabby body and waist, even if you weigh and measure less, is but a camouflage to a fatter body. Your body is smaller only because it has shrunk—or atrophied. Your heart muscle, the muscles of your arteries and the muscles of your digestive system have withered from lack of enough use. You have a poison-filled, acidosis-saturated body. When you aren't active enough or don't do enough systematic exercise, your legs turn flabby. So will your body and waistline.

One of the principal needs for healthy thighs and calves is vitamin C. Vitamin C is also an important contributor to a trim body and a small waist. Your legs need vitamin C because it strengthens the inner walls of their capillaries. The pull of gravity drags your circulating blood down into your legs and feet, and you need strong capillaries, arteries and veins to receive this blood and pump it back to your lungs and heart. If they can't do it effectively, you have to limit your activity or you will tire easily from lack of enough oxygen in your blood. Fat then accumulates faster on your body and around your waist. To counteract this evil through fasting, pills or fad diets may help you "thin down" again. But you will turn flabby through lessened activity, and you will atrophy with increasing debility into premature old age.

Your thighs and legs also depend significantly upon the strength of their bones. Your lower limbs consist mostly of muscle supported by bone, and they bear the whole weight of your body when you stand or move on your feet. They are at rest only when you sit or lie down. Vitamin C is essential to your bone development. (So are vitamins A and D).

HOW TO NATURALLY GET THE LEGS-STRENGTHENING VITAMIN YOU NEED

The best sources of vitamin C are citrus fruits and tomatoes. Other natural sources may be richer, but they are either inedible or can't be eaten in large quantities. Green peppers and parsley, for example, contain more vitamin C than oranges, but you are not likely to eat enough of them. Spinach and other greens also contain appreciable amounts of vitamin C, but they lose it progressively when stored at room temperatures. But citrus fruit and tomato juice lose it only slightly, even when canned. The vitamin C contents of cantaloupes, strawberries, cabbage and turnips, when raw, just about equal that of tomatoes. Potatoes, fresh peas, asparagus and lettuce are excellent sources. Liver is the best animal source. Fish roe and milt (spleen) are also rich in it. Other sources are cherries (but they are soaked with dyes), apples, cashew apple, Cuban fruits, honey, watercress, broccoli, rose hips (perhaps the richest source, and it hasn't the enamel-eroding citric acid of citrus fruits), sprouted soybeans (but they take a lot of time and space to prepare), watermelons, raw cabbage, collards and turnip greens (but they are full of spray). My high intake of fruits, citrus fruits, pineapples and potatoes in my diet has kept me well supplied with vitamin C. Although I oppose IQ tests, a Texas study shows that children with a higher level of ascorbic acid in the blood averaged five points higher in the IQ than those with low levels.

But, you have to prevent all sources of vitamin C from coming into contact with air over a long period of time, because they lose the vitamin through oxidation. But that is not the worst effect. When oxidized, vitamin C is diabetogenic (it may cause diabetes). Being ascorbic acid, vitamin C is converted by oxidation into dehydroascorbic acid: an acid that destroys the sulphydryl groups of enzymes essential to the use of sugar (carbohydrate) by your body. Since garlic also contains a sulphydryl group of enzymes (SH), oxidized vitamin C would inactivate its powerful beneficial effects. *Note*: The sulphydryl group of enzymes in garlic must therefore also help the body use its sugar and decrease the severity of diabetes. This observation of mine may turn out to be another miracle discovery.

HOW TO EAT CITRUS FRUITS AND PROTECT YOUR TEETH FROM THEM

The best way to eat citrus fruits, it would seem, would be to eat the whole fruit. That is how most authorities suggest to eat it. Doing so, though, implants your teeth for some time into the citric acid in the juice as well as into that within the pulp. Tooth erosion is then inescapable. Here is a much safer way which I have developed and used for years.

1. Slice the citrus fruit in half and squeeze out the juice with a hand squeezer. Wear a cloth working glove, to prevent your hand from absorbing the insecticides on the skin of the fruit. Cover the juice immediately to reduce the consequent vitamin C oxidation as much as possible.
2. Strain the juice to remove the pulp. Then
3. Dilute the juice with about an equal volume of water.
4. The pulp of citrus fruit is rich with vitamin A. But it is soaked with citrus juice. So, place it in a small container and cover it with water. Squash it with a ladle to squeeze out all the juice. Strain this water through a strainer and add it to the juice.

5. Hold the strainer containing the pulp under running water and squash out any remaining citrus juice. The pulp will have lost all its juice by now and should be taken to the table and eaten like a vegetable.
6. Drink the juice when you are about halfway through your meal. Draw it down through a straw to keep the juice away from your teeth. Don't try to mix it with saliva, or it will linger too long in your mouth. After every long sip or two, chew a piece of banana to keep the juice from coming into contact with your teeth. Once the glass is empty, chew at least half a banana to absorb all the juice which remains in your mouth, mixed with saliva.

That's how I eat citrus fruit. Make sure it does *not* taste acrid when you suck it down. The procedure takes about 7 minutes, but I value citrus fruits highly.

(Tangerines are excepted. Peel and eat them whole because they contain too little eroding citric acid to imperil your tooth enamel).

WHY YOU SHOULD NOT GIVE UP ON CITRUS FRUITS

Although I have nothing against rose-hips, I am convinced that citrus fruits possess a not-yet-discovered youth extender which scientists do not suspect. The pulp of citrus fruits is also an unsurpassed natural laxative and efficiently balances your weight. That's why I don't replace them with other rich vitamin C foods like rose-hips.

Caution: Don't cut and eat the citrus fruit unless it feels soft enough to your touch. When it is still hard it is green, overacid and contains less vitamin C than it should.

I don't recommend vitamin C pills because the citric or ascorbic acid (or both) in them is so tart that it "burns" (or at least irritates) the inner lining of your urinary bladder. When repeated over a period of time, such irritations may lead to undesirable consequences. To determine the amount of vitamin C quantitatively in blood or urine, a dye (sodium 2,6-dichlorobenzenone indophenol) is injected under the skin and forms a blue spot. If no ascorbic acid (vitamin C) is present, the blue spot remains. The more vitamin C there is in the tissues, the faster the blue spot disappears. Vitamin C, in brief, is a bleach. Should you take too much of it, as you are likely to do with any concentrated preparation, it must bleach your insides a bit. That's why I believe that it can irritate the linings of your kidneys, bladder and urethra.

THE SECRET OF THE POWER-HOUSE FOODS

Probably no other food can provide your calves and thighs with their unusual strength better than nuts. Nuts fill your whole body with unmatched stamina. With them, you can be unusually active day-after-day and stay trim with your waist down. But they should be combined with other foods because they lack certain vitamins and minerals which are found in large quantities in other foods. Most nuts contain plenty of phosphorus. Phosphorus is important in your daily nourishment, and you get lots of it from cereals, legumes, nuts and food of animal origin, like meat and eggs. To assimilate and use it properly, however, you need much calcium in your food at the same time, and you assimilate the calcium with vitamin D, the sunshine vitamin. Nuts abound in iron, and your blood needs iron to transport the oxygen you inhale to your tissues. It also needs it to transport the carbon dioxide waste in your tissues to your lungs to be exhaled. Without enough iron in your blood you become anemic, fatigue easily when active or exercising and become flabby.

Nuts contain much magnesium. Your blood vessels are kept toned by magnesium. They may dilate otherwise, and your blood then forms pools in your splanchnic (your visceral, abdominal) blood vessels, and you are plunged into lassitude and torpitude. Your food loses magnesium when it is refined. Magnesium is in whole grain flour, for example, but not in white flour. It is also in brown rice but not in white rice. Lack of enough phosphorus in your food adds to your magnesium-caused lethargy, because phosphorus is an important ingredient of brain tissue. Lack of enough of it in your food turns you slow and pessimistic, and you avoid activity with your legs all you can and lose your body trimness and small waist even faster.

THE YOUTH-BRINGING MIRACLE OF CERTAIN FOODS

Nuts, best of all, are packed with vitamin B and E. You need vitamin B for the health of your nerves. Nerve power makes you active, which keeps you trim. You are unusually tired and under unnecessary tension otherwise. You abhor the daily effort of an occupation and still more that of healthy physical exercise. (Vitamin E will be discussed later in this chapter).

As with vegetables and fruits, though, most nuts lack one or more of the essential amino acids, or they contain some of them in such small quantities that your body can't utilize them to build up the protein in your tissues fast enough to save you from atrophying much sooner than you should. Every succeeding day of your life, you naturally atrophy closer to old age and death. You can delay it remarkably by reversing it as much as possible. But even peanut flour and soybean flour, which abound in most of the amino acids, are deficient in two most important ones, the cholesterol-ridding methionine and the cataract-preventing tryptophane. Yet, unless you consume *all* the essential amino acids you need *at the same meal*, the protein you eat does you little good. The amino acids which it does contain *won't wait* in your digestive tract for the missing ones. But proteins are the building blocks of your body. They keep you being and looking young by delaying the inevitable atrophy of living long. So, keep on reading.

THE FOOD FOR MENTAL AND PHYSICAL POWER

If you are a vegetarian, but don't exclude eggs or any other form of animal protein, you will retard immensely the atrophying process of aging. Milk and eggs add vitamin B_{12} to the vegetables, wiich contain none. Your whole grain cereals contain protein, but they have less and less because the soils are wearing out faster then they can be rebuilt. That's why you have to add the Triple Tonic Secret to your eating, or risk the uncertainties of taking food supplements and concentrated food pills. Nuts provide another unsurpassed nutritional advantage for keeping you "eternally young" and trim (and, of course, small-waisted). They are far less affected by the use of strong chemicals than the leaves of the stalks, and therefore contain far more minerals. A mineral like phosphorus, which is found in fish, is believed to be a brain stimulant. Nuts contain 20 to 21 times more phosphorus than fish. Animals that are fed raw grain seeds (nuts) perform much more work than those who graze pasture alone. So, nuts fill you with *both* mental *and* physical power.

THAT certainly amounts to prolonging your youth! That's what keeps you active, toned up and willing to exercise enough to make your body *solidly* trim and keep your waist *firmly* small. Both of these do much to keep your weight ideal.

HOW TO PRESERVE THE MIRACLE POWER OF YOUTH-BRINGING FOODS

Never eat nuts roasted, salted or in any other form than raw. Eat them at the end or near the end of your meal, for most of them contain a respectable percentage of unsaturated fatty acids. All fat compounds digest the slowest of all foods. Don't chew nuts. They are too solid, and the trauma of breaking them down fine with your teeth erodes your enamel. Grind them down before each meal and let them soak in milk, to soften still more. Your teeth and gums don't have to be traumatized by your food, as so many preach, to be strong. Such unnecessary hard chewing wears out your teeth early, and you can't chew nuts effectively with false teeth. Hard chewing also brings on gingivitis instead of strengthening your gums. *Never* crack nuts or their shells with your teeth. Leave that for the squirrels. I have known boxers who tried to toughen their jaws by hammering them with their own fists, or by letting their sparring partners batter their jaws for them. They ended up punch-drunk and easy knockout victims of their opponents. Don't eat too many nuts at one time either. A flat, level handful once a day is sufficient. *Never* eat nuts between meals. In fact, eat *nothing* between meals. (This is discussed thoroughly later).

Don't engage in unusual bending, twisting, speedy movements, much less in moderate or strenuous exercise for three hours after eating nuts. Nuts are concentrated food. Their oils and unsaturated fatty acids digest slowly compared to the pectin of fruits and the fibers of vegetables. They fill you with energy and "stay" with you a long time; but you can't hurry their digestion. When you try to, you bloat your "belly" with gas and look shapeless. You disrupt your digestion, rob your body of nutriment and deprive your muscles of the repair they need to remain active at work or in exercise. In time, you will suffer from indigestion headaches on the top and left side of your head, frown in discomfort and look surly and antisocial. Eat nuts wisely and feel strong in your legs. You will restrain, for decades, the ever-encroaching atrophy of the years and look and feel young and stay trim with a teen-age waist.

FOODS THAT ATTACK CHOLESTEROL AND MAKE YOU TRIM

You won't have a trim body and a small, firm waist if your cholesterol level is high. The long-lived people of the world's Shangri-las spend most of their days climbing up and down the rugged terrain where they live, to "earn their daily bread." They have little time left to lie around and reminisce about getting old and complain about their different aches and pains. And they have very few. No fast-food diet, vitamin pills, supplements, food concentrate or food substitutes can bring you their bones and joints and free you from weakened hips or feet as you advance in years. Their weights and waists remain normal without their even trying. Their waists could be smaller and shapelier if they did the Abdominal Double Curl, but they don't aspire to look like fashion models. One of the foremost results of their way of life is that it reduces their cholesterol levels to such a degree that many claim to be 150 years old or more.

In the "advanced" areas where you live, you can't live like those people. Besides, you don't have the time or the inclination. And yet, when your legs feel young, you feel young all over, and your body stays trim and your waist stays small. So, you do whatever exercise you can and add dietary aids to get stronger legs and reduce your cholesterol level. "Sex foods" or vitamins are important aids in this connection. Estrogen (the female sex vitamin) lowers your blood cholesterol. That's why vitamin E, the "sex vitamin," has been demonstrated in the laboratory to slow down aging. Wheat germ oil, which is rich in vitamin E, reduces your waist and hips and builds up your muscles (which includes your leg muscles, the biggest and most used muscles of your body). When you take wheat germ oil regularly you feel euphoric, tireless, and light in body, as if walking on air. You feel likewise from taking high-protein pills, anabolic steroids and megavitamins.

But They are not Strictly Natural

None of these sources of vitamins, hormones or amino acids, however, are strictly natural. High-proteins and megavitamins implant too much of certain food substances into your system and abuse your different organs. They overburden your liver in its efforts to detoxify their excess concentrations, strain your kidneys as they strive to filter the excess acids they excrete, and which "burn" the linings of their blood filtering tubules. Since you cannot maintain whatever benefits you derive from these excessive concentrations unless you continue then indefinitely, even if you lessen them, your traumatized organs risk eventual suffering from irreversible damages.

Wheat germ oil, or any other concentration of vitamin E, and anabolic steroids, may cause massive hormonal changes in your body which bring about fantastic changes in you. They overstimulate certain glands in your body to secrete more of their hormones than they do normally. To "fool around" with your glands is not to be recommended. When overstimulated long enough they could start overgrowing on their own.

THE TWO NATURAL WAYS TO INCREASE YOUR SEX POWER AND THE STRENGTH IN YOUR LEGS

It is safer to limit yourself to the natural foods which contain vitamin E (the "sex vitamin") and increase their effectiveness with the Triple Tonic Secret without artificially overstimulating your glands. I have proved it in myself and in many followers. Here is the secret. Your body synthesizes about 10 times your daily intake of cholesterol per day. When you increase your dietary intake of cholesterol, your body automatically forms less of it. You therefore *don't have* to take estrogen-like substances to decrease the cholesterol content of your blood. You just have to follow one or two dietary directions. These are:

1. *The Food Limiting Direction.* Eat less food containing saturated fats, and thereby reduce your daily calorie intake. (You happen to do this to a maximum when you fast). Simultaneously, eat more foods containing vitamin E. In other words, eat more fruits and vegetables, but also eat more eggs (two a day for a while), more leafy green vegetables, beans and grains. One of the essential amino acids is arginine. In an arginine-deficient diet, seminal fluid shows a reduction in the number of spermatozoa. Eighty percent of the sperm protein consists of arginine. When arginine is added to the diet, the number of sperm cells is restored to normal.[1] In the young chick a deficiency causes profound weakness and reduced muscle creatine content. (Creatine is involved in muscle metabolism). Don't fail to eat foods containing this essential amino acid, arginine, both for sex power and leg muscle strength. The two go together.

I have made a list of the most easily procured sources of arginine, in the order of their greatest unit content. Tigernut (950), tropical almond (919), hazelnut (864-975), coconut (dried kernel (822), walnut (725-812), sesame (756), buckwheat (613), pea (595), chicken-pea (588), cabbage (519), wheat germ (513), yam (477), banana (469), cucumber (469), egg yolk (469), grape (460), fish (cod, haddock) (412), catfish (405), brussel sprouts (356-405). Some foreign foods contain the most: Ethiopian marvolanut (988), African mammee-apple (981), tacca (Fiji-arrowroot) 869.[2]

The sperm count in an individual with "idiopathic hypospermia" (reduced sperm count without change in the sperm synthesizing apparatus) was increased several fold by administering 8 grams of arginine per day.

2. *The Triple Tonic Secret Direction.* This is the second direction to reduce the cholesterol content of your blood without taking estrogen-like substances. Your body synthesizes about 10 times your daily intake of cholesterol. If you could reduce this amount of synthesis you would have little to worry about how much cholesterol you ate in your food. You can reduce it with the Triple Tonic Secret. This is how. Many tissues in your body synthesize cholesterol. These include your adrenals, testes (man), ovaries (woman), small intestine, skin and muscle (smaller amounts). But your liver is the most important site. Your plasma (blood) cholesterol comes chiefly from your liver. Slow down your "regeneration time", or the time you require to synthesize an amount of cholesterol equal to the amount present in your body. Your regeneration time for plasma cholesterol is about 12 days, and your daily synthesis seems to be about 500 to 600 mg. per day. (Tittenberg) The Triple Tonic Secret consists of slowing down to an undiagnosable degree the "regeneration time" of your cholesterol in your liver and in speeding up the activity of your thyroids. When the thyroid is overactive, the concentration of cholesterol in the blood is decreased.

Your sex power and the strength in your legs will increase surprisingly. It is revealed in Illustration 14.

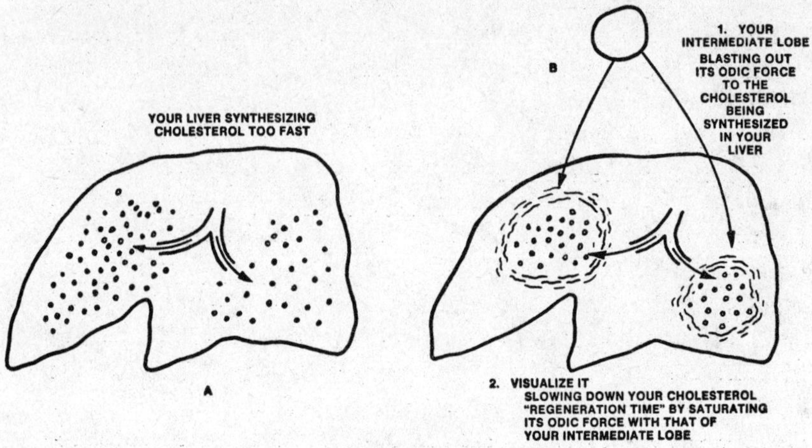

Illustration 14

How Lena R. Became a Sylph-Like Tigress in Her Sport Activity

Lena R. aspired to excel in her sport but lacked enough agility to compete against the respected performers. No matter how hard she trained and tried in competition, she never made the grade.

With the *Yogatronic Diet* Lena lost about nine pounds of hard-to-remove weight in about five weeks, and about an inch from her waist. Her legs felt more springy, her reach longer, her movements faster and her flexibility greater. She slipped more easily into her best vantage points and made her best moves more spontaneously. Her endurance increased remarkably, and she outlasted rival after rival. Her victories became consistent, and she started training for the big events, confident of reaching the top. She called the Triple Tonic Secret "a miracle."

How Anita Q. Captured a Wealthy Stranger for a Husband

Anita Q.'s main worry about her attraction was her thighs. She could conceal them in skirts but not in bathing suits. She tried different exercises, but they didn't help enough, and she couldn't spend "all day exercising." She begged me to help her.

With the *Yogatronic Diet* Anita lost from nine to 12 pounds of stubborn weight in four weeks. But she retained her vim and vitality to be active and still exercise. The fiber in her food carried out much of the food fat and thinned her thighs. The arginine-containing foods increased her sex appeal. In a few months her thighs slimmed down delightfully, and she was charged with more energy and exercised more vigorously. A wealthy stranger joined her in her favorite sport—and married her.

REFERENCES

[1]Holt, L.E., and Najjar, V.A. Proc. Fed/Am. Soc. Exp. Biol., 1942.

[2]"*Amino-Acid Content of Foods and Biological Data on Proteins*." Food and Agriculture Organization of the United Nations. Food Policy and Food Science Service, Nutrition Division, FAO. Second Printing, 1972. Rome, Italy.

16

how yogatronics gives you attention-getting hips—effortlessly

THE MOST CRUCIAL SUPPORTING STRUCTURE OF YOUR BODY

Whether you are a man or a woman, you won't have a trim figure and a small waist unless your hips are strong, healthy and shapely. The long-lived people of the world's Shangri-las have strong, normally functioning hip-joints, or they could not daily climb up and down the rugged terrains on which they live. Without strong healthy hips you can't be as active as you should and are confined to much sitting or lying down, both of which weaken your hips and fatten you still more. Old people's hips in our civilized world are usually so weak that they fracture easily. If they are not too advanced in years, their weak hips can be surgically replaced, but even after that, they have to be active, or fat and cholesterol accumulate in them and shorten their lives.

Besides, whether you are a man or a woman, your hips can make or break the symmetry of your figure. They are located, more or less, in the exact center of your body, and unless they are maintained in proportion to your sex and figure, they distort your whole appearance. When they "fit" with your figure, they add immeasurably to its appeal. They also have to match your waist. When you trim your waist your hips look bigger. They have to be trimmed, too, or they detract from your improved figure. If you are a man, trim hips bring you a more youthful look. Your shoulders look broader, and your height seems taller. Your hips can be rounder and fuller if you are a woman; but don't let them spread or your shoulders will "narrow" and your legs "thin" by comparison. But if they are too flat and narrow, they might not look feminine enough to many a man. Keep them as slender as possible, nonetheless, for they are inclined to fill out and broaden with time, even if your remain active or exercise.

EATING HABITS THAT BRING ON EVER-THREATENING BOTTOM SPREAD

Carbohydrates are your energy-giving food. If their energy is not used up, they are deposited as fat in certain fat depots of your body, such as your waist or hips. Sugar is the carbohydrate you consume most of, and it is the main dietary enemy of your hips. It does not maintain your health, and you can't stay healthy with enlarging hips because they are a sign that you are eating too much sugar, too much fat or not being sufficiently active. Sugar does not build up your body or repair your tissues, as proteins do. Neither does it take part, like proteins and fats, in many of your complex body processes. You won't feel driven to be active enough, on the other hand, without its energy to feed your efforts. You will fatten in body and waist, become constipated and lose your figure and health. But when your hips "spread", it indicates that you sit too much, your bowels don't move completely enough, your waist is bulging or starting to, your trunk is sagging downwards, your visceral organs (including your heart) are being compressed from above and below and have less room and blood supply to function properly.

Your bio-rhythm is thrown out of gear, you develop vague discomforts and even nagging headaches, you feel your age—or much older than you are. You are eating too much carbohydrate either because you have a "sweet tooth" or because of a snack-eating habit. Snacks, or eating between meals, is the surest way to fatten your hips (your waist and your whole body), ruin your digestion and your liver and curse you with constipation and diverticulitis. The very fact that you ought to wait for each snack to digest before you become energetically active permits your body to accumulate more fat than it would otherwise.

FOODS THAT RUIN YOUR HIPS AND YOUR YOUTHFUL SHAPE

Here is a list of foods that contain different percentages of figure-ruining sugar.

1. Foods with five percent sugar, which fatten your hips the least, are: carrots, cauliflower, okra, onions, peppers, pumpkin, radishes, string beans and watercress.
2. Foods with about seven percent sugar are: grapefruit, lemons, strawberries, watermelon. So are avocados and olives, but they are quite high in fat and won't keep your hips thin unless you exercise long or strenuously.
3. Foods with 10 percent sugar, which will add weight on you unless you dissipate their extra energy in enough activity or exercise, are: parsnips, peas, Hubbard squash, turnips, berries, cantaloupe, muskmelon, oranges, peaches, pineapple, raspberries.
4. Foods with 15 percent sugar, which require strenuous or long activity or exercise to use up the energy they deposit in your body, are: apples, apricots, cherries, currants, grapes, huckleberries, nectarines, pears. (The skins of many of these foods are thickly coated with insecticides, so don't eat too many of them at one meal). Eat raw garlic on such days to extract their poisons from your cells. Add the Triple Tonic Secret (page 49) to counteract it further.
5. Foods with about 25 percent sugar, which tend to fatten your hips and waist (and whole body) unless you exercise strenuously, jog 1-1/2 hours a day or climb many flights of steps regularly, are: corn, lima beans, navy beans, sweet and white potatoes, rice, bananas, fresh figs, plums and prunes. Dried fruits fatten your hips much more, for they contain as much as 75 percent sugar (or carbohydrate).

   Sugar peas contain the most sugar when the pea is too

immature to be eaten, but they lose considerable vitamins after picking. Their sugar content lessens, but their starch content increases. I have eaten them all my life and am surviving excellently with this depleted stable food. Thanks to the Triple Tonic Secret at the end of this chapter.

HOW OVERINDULGENCE IN SEX ALTERS THE SHAPE OF YOUR HIPS AND YOUR FIGURE

Activity is most important for your hips, for it has been long established[1] that exercise causes your body to use more vitamins. Rodale (and I agree with him) proposes that this is probably the result of better oxygenation and improved digestion that results, I assume he means, from the healthy strain of exercise on the body. Months earlier[2] the *Journal of the American Medical Association* announced that "the greatest value of exercise" was that it stimulated your endocrine glands, particularly your thyroid, to greater activity. Your endocrine glands slow down with age and contribute to old age fatigue (Rodale). That's why you need strong hips all your life, or your period of youth is abbreviated the moment they turn weak. Even prostate disease, which occurs in 60 percent of men, is partly the result of lack of exercise. Dr. John Nesfield, in the *British Medical Journal*,[3] announced that prostate trouble is commonplace in "pampered house dogs," but not in "working" dogs like foxhounds, farm dogs and sheepdogs.

If you are a man, the acidity of your semen is about the same as that of your blood. Your semen has a lower concentration of chloride and cholesterol than your blood, but it has a higher concentration of phosphorus and lactic acid. The purpose of its high phosphorus content (phosphate) is undoubtedly to buffer any acid in the secretion of your mate. Your semen has about twice the concentration of calcium, urea and sugar of your blood. The sugar in it is fructose (fruit sugar), rather than glucose. It is therefore absorbed more slowly than the sugar in your blood. The competing athlete who has not indulged in sex for weeks previous to a contest carries a reservoir of energy "below his belt" to draw upon in decisive moments. It explains why overindulgence in sex, if you are a man, depletes your sugar (glycogen) reserve by drawing more glucose from your blood to convert to fructose in your semen. You suffer from a mild fatigue, as a consequence, exercise less, get heavier and bigger waisted.

LITTLE GHOSTS IN YOU THAT ENABLE YOUR FOOD TO MAKE YOU STRONG

Your hips will not be strong if the food you eat does not make you as strong as it can, and it won't if the enzymes in your digestive tract and in your metabolic processes are not potent enough. Enzymes are not foods. They are substances in your food and in you that trigger necessary chemical changes in your food so that it can be absorbed and assimilated. Enzymes have the unusual quality of causing chemical changes without heat. Like unseen ghosts, they possess the miracle power to stimulate specific chemical changes without contributing *any* energy of their own. That's why an enzyme is called a "catalyst." It remains *absolutely unchanged* in the midst of the most violent changes it causes in you or your food. It acts like a ghost drifting through a violent human scene it has brought about. That's why it can cause miracles to happen in you with your food.

Its activity, however, can be halted by cold or heat. Enzymes trigger the reactions faster with a small increase of heat, but they are destroyed with more heat, even after the food mixture is cooled. They are very active between 32 and 104 degrees Farhenheit. When heated above 122° F., they are permanently annihilated. You also destroy them when you roast meat at 200° or 300°F.

That's why your refrigerator is such a valuable appliance. When you keep foods like lettuce, celery and radishes at room temperature, they wither because their enzymes remain active at that temperature and continue triggering aging chemical reactions in them. When you store these foods in the refrigerator, their enzymes hibernate and the foods stop aging and stay fresh. It proves that the aging process, whether in man, plant or animal, *can* be halted, as *Yogatronics* accomplishes.

How The Little Food-Ghosts Work

Only a modicum of enzymes are needed to trigger a chemical reaction in your body. Every one of your cells contains enzymes, and your body has several billion cells. Your enzymes are the only connection your cells have with the rest of your body. Your salivary glands, your pancreas, your stomach and your intestines contain your main digestive enzymes, which number up to nine. This is most significant because the vitamins in your food can operate *only* when enzymes are present in your digestive juices. Each vitamin forms, with particular enzymes, complex enzyme systems. Every vitamin in your body, for that reason, is a part of an enzyme system.

Your body never gets hot enough to destroy its enzyme systems. Some enzymes, in addition, work only in an acid medium like your stomach. Other enzymes need an alkaline medium, like your intestines. For example, when you are sick or your stomach is not well, your stomach won't secrete enough hydrochloric acid to digest your food. Your proteins won't digest in your stomach (the site of their digestion) because your ill stomach lacks enough pepsin, the enzyme in it that triggers protein digestion. Pepsin triggers protein digestion in an acid stomach but not in an alkaline one. That's why drinking water when you eat meat, slows down the digestion of the meat in your stomach. The water turns your stomach alkaline. As you grow older you digest meat (protein) less completely because your stomach secretes less hydrochloric acid. That's why, at the end of this chapter, you will be taught how to defy old age by keeping your stomach young with the Triple Tonic Secret.

RAW FOODS AND ENZYMES

Raw foods contain enzymes, but cooking destroys the enzymes. The amount of enzymes your body needs to digest cooked food is, consequently, far more than it needs to digest raw food. Raw food contains far more enzymes than cooked food, which help your body digest it. Eating raw food overworks your digestive glands (like overworking the glands of your pancreas when you digest starchy foods) far less than cooked food. It explains why you feel full faster with raw food, unless you season the cooked food and fool yourself into thinking that you have eaten your fill, when you are actually only half nourished. Hence, you either overeat when you eat cooked food because "it tastes so nice" or you undereat and think you are full. So, you either fatten your hips, your waist and your whole body, or you weaken yourself and become less active, more flabby and lose your symmetry.

How To Get the Most Enzyme Power Out of Your Food

To get the most benefit out of raw food and keep your hips slim, you ought to grate or shred most of your raw food. Never cook fruits, except just enough to soften the hard dried ones, like figs. Frozen fruit retains its enzymes, but should be eaten as soon as it thaws. Don't eat it cold. Cold inactivates the enzymes, so that cold food passes through you undigested.

Enzymes are proteins. They are destroyed easily by heat, because proteins change when heated. Food digestion is most important to the strength of your hips (to your whole body) because it both builds up and breaks down your tissues. It causes your cells to breathe and stay alive, and permits your muscles to contract more fully by supplying them with nutrition. You possess your own pattern of enzyme efficiency, however. It is difficult to explain by logic, but your physiological, mental and psychic realms exert controlling influence over it. Your enzyme efficiency might vary with that of your neighbor or companion not by a mere 20 to 50 percent, but more often by at least two to four-fold. In a substantial number of cases, you and other "normal" people might differ by 10 to 50-fold. The details of the complete metabolisms of you and your neighbor, even if both of you are diagnosed as normal in the clinic, might vary 10-fold. The cause baffles material science because material science has not given full importance to the grip of your mind over the food you eat. Learn how to use the Triple Tonic Secret to recreate or replenish enough of the enzymes which the food you eat has lost through the evils involved in the raising, handling and storing of modern civilization. It will be a big help to keep your hips slim, healthy and strong—and it will keep your waist small, and your weight ideal. (See Illus. 15 for this Triple Tonic Secret).

How Alma W. to Her Amusement, Suddenly Was Offered a Job as a "Stripper"

All her life Alma W. had been angry at the size of her hips. They ruined her proportions. She was too lazy to be very active or

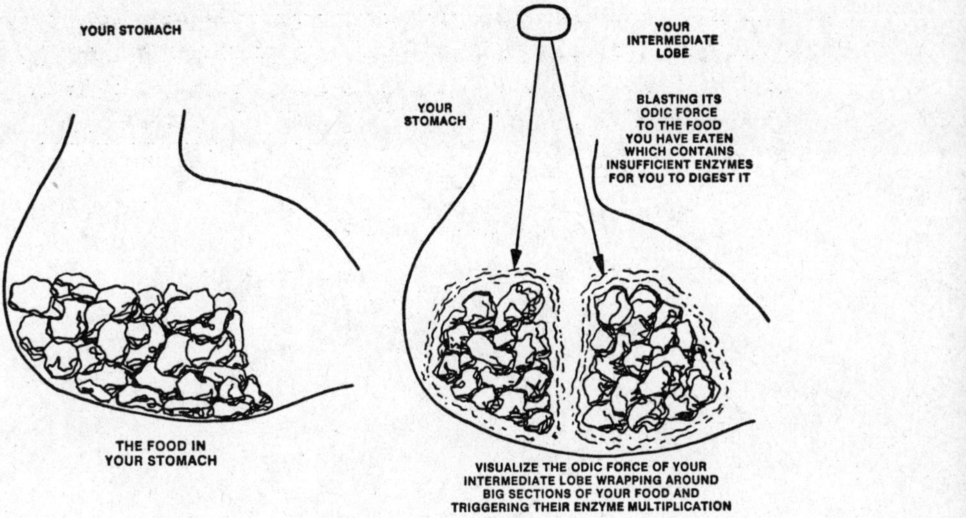

Illustration 15

to do much exercise, and that bulked her hips still more. But she yearned to look like females with attractive hips.

With the *Yogatronic Diet* and the ending of snacks, Alma lost 15 pounds in six weeks from the fat deposits of her waist, hips and thighs. The Triple Tonic Secret, she raved, speeded it up like magic. Shortly thereafter, her figure looked so sensational to the eye that she was offered a high-paying job as a strip-tease dancer—at which she giggled.

How Archie R. Was Unexpectedly Selected for the High Position He Wanted

Archie R. was more industrious than anyone he knew, but he was repeatedly passed by for the position he craved. He fared no better romantically and was "disgusted with everything."

I perceived, at a glance, that his overweight hips distorted his appearance. They ruined his symmetry, "shortened" his height, sheared him of elegance, and robbed him of the appearance of being able to manage others. Despite his tested ability and knowledge in his occupation, his shapeless hips (and his enlarged waist, which accompanied them) failed to impress his superiors easily.

With the *Yogatronic Diet* and The Abdominal Double Curl,

Archie's hips and waist shrank with surprising speed, and his attitude changed before he even realized it. With the Triple Tonic Secret his hips "thinned down while eating." He felt as if he were gliding across the ground instead of walking. Within six months, he was promoted, at last, to the position he had coveted for a decade.

REFERENCES

[1]*Journal of Nutrition*, April 10, 1958.
[2]*Journal of the American Medical Association*, October 5, 1957.
[3]Dr. John Nesfield, in the *British Medical Journal*, January 19, 1957.

17

yogatronic secrets for firming your arms and holding them to the right size

WHY YOUR ARMS ARE IMPORTANT FOR CONTROLLING YOUR WEIGHT AND THE SIZE OF YOUR WAIST

Whether you are a man or woman, it is difficult to be masterful and have a trim body and a small waist when your arms lack tone. Your arms need not be ropey with muscle, but they should not be blubbery with fat or flabby with thinness. Your whole body, in fact, should be toned up with your arms, or you will lack the incentive to be active or to exercise enough to maintain your arms firm. Using your muscles causes your body to produce an unusual amount of heat. That's why you burn off calories when you are active or exercise. But use of your muscles won't cause you to lose weight or acquire a thin waist unless your body gets warm in the process. Ordinarily, muscle work increases the temperature of your body from 0.1 to 1° F. Soon after you stop, your body temperature returns to normal. Consequently, if you want to lose weight rapidly you also have to consume less of certain kinds of foods, even if you are quite active or engage in exercise.

Furthermore, you can lose weight with activity or exercises, only if you throw large groups of muscles into severe and rather prolonged contractions simultaneously. In marathon races, body temperatures of 104° F. have been recorded. Such an increase in body heat also increases the speed of your breathing and heart beat and is therefore beneficial to your lungs and heart, providing that you exert yourself within your normal capacity.

ONE OF THE BEST WAYS TO LOSE WEIGHT

You cannot control your weight by exercising your arms alone. One of the best ways to lose weight is to eat foods containing certain vitamins like vitamin E. Wheat germ oil contains abundant vitamin E. Taking it is a sure way to reduce. The same is true of the hormone of the thyroid gland. These two "foods" throw you into euphoria by making you feel so "light," but they do so by overstimulating your sex or your thyroid glands, which is something I cannot recommend freely. I prefer to take buttermilk, yogurt or acidophilus milk. The fermented milk of the last two contains tremendous amounts of lactic acid-producing bacteria, which tend to replace your intestinal bacteria. Dry skim milk will not fatten you either. Neither of these milks will weaken you and limit your daily activity or physical efforts. They don't leave you feeling as abnormally euphoric as wheat germ oil or thyroid pills, because they don't overstimulate your endocrine glands. They are therefore safe, but they will limit your weight and keep your arms trim and good-looking or make them big and muscular if you exercise for power.

CERTAIN DRAWBACKS ABOUT MILK

Note: It is a pity that practically all milk now contains traces of penicillin. The cow is given penicillin to prevent or cure disease. Milk is also deficient in one of the essential amino acids. Concentrated or dried milk loses vitamin A, too, because the vitamin is heat-liable, but you can make up for that loss by eating carrots. Milk is an excellent food for an adult. Its proteins are among the best, and its carbohydrate and fat are digested and assimilated easily. One quart of milk daily provides you with more than the usual calcium you require, with two-thirds of the phosphorus and with a full amount of riboflavin (vitamin B_2). Milk's leading drawback is its low iron content. Eat raisins to make up for it. Raisins, however, contain much sulphur, so don't consume too many of them at one sitting. I myself, though, have eaten milk, eggs and raisins daily for seven-eights of my life, and I am bursting with good health. I do not justify the consumption of poisoned food, but my taking raw garlic regularly plus using the Triple Tonic Secret seem to have protected me effectively against the perils of store food consumption in our civilized society.

HOW TO BE ABLE TO EAT LESS SUGAR AND LOSE WEIGHT EASIER

Much of the sugar in you is used up during muscular activity or during exposure to cold. You respond by eating more sugar than you should. Prevent this by being sweet-natured when you are active or exercising. It is not easy to do so, but that's how you can calm your sympathetic nervous system and reduce your muscles' call for sugar. Violent emotions, like fear and rage, use up your stored sugar. If you are very active or engage in demanding exercise, your fear and rage will deplete your sugar stores all the more, will abnormally increase your appetite for sugar and will fatten you and enlarge your waist. With the Triple Tonic Secret (Illus. 16), control the quantity of sugar your body demands at such times and lose weight much easier without fasting or curbing your appetite. Your arms will become just as strong but will be trimmer. In sports and even at work, you tire less easily by staying cool in the midst of action.

FOODS THAT ADD STRENGTH TO YOUR ARMS AND BODY

Spinach has been praised for a long time as a food that makes you strong. When you are strong, you can be trim and have a small firm waist. Spinach is rich in vitamin C, and it contains almost as much vitamin A as carrots. It has an abundance of vitamin B and calcium and three times the quantity of iron found in carrots and potatoes. Unfortunately, it also contains oxalic acid (expecially in its

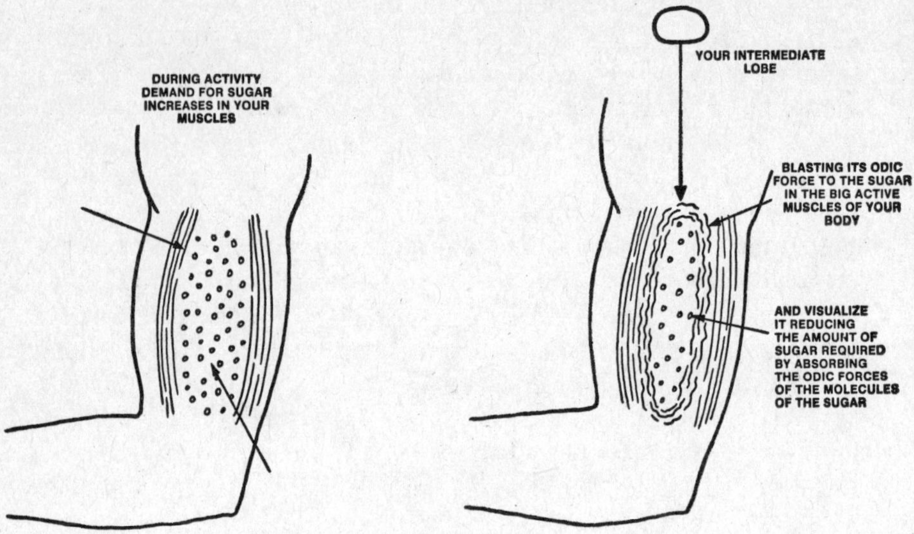

Illustration 16

young tender sprigs), which combines with calcium and robs your body of it. Yet, you need calcium, because among other things, it keeps your system from turning too acid or alkaline and makes the energy in your food available for your muscles.

Excess fat in your food contains no oxalic acid, but it reduces your body's absorption of calcium, although a small amount of fat in your food improves your body's absorption of calcium.

Other foods whose content of oxalic acid rob your body of calcium, particularly when you consume several of them at one meal, are: rhubarb, beet leaves, cocoa, tea, chocolate, candy, sorrel, figs, potatoes, beans (navy), string beans, cabbage, gooseberries, plums, endive, strawberries, tomatoes, beets, celery, bread and grapefruit. Oats robs your calcium, too, with their phytic acid The calcium is robbed from your food in the lumen, the hollow space in your gut-tube, and rendered unavailable for absorption through its walls. To counteract this steady drain of your food calcium, you have to take more whole milk, soybeans, beef liver, eggs, cabbage (although it contains much oxalic acid) and turnips. A good source of calcium is turnip greens, but they are also thickly coated with sprays, so I don't recommend them.

For arm and body power, eat carbohydrates with fats such as fruits with nuts. Such a combination adds 50 percent or more to your calories and spares your proteins. It reduces the amount of sugar you have to eat to get the energy to build up your muscles and firm up your arms.

THE MAGIC FOOD FOR YOUR BLOOD

Your blood should be thick enough (containing enough hemoglobin in its red blood corpuscles) to transport adequate supplies of oxygen to your organs and muscles. Bananas keep it thick enough because the iron in them is in a chemical form which can be used to form hemoglobin. Bananas also spare much of your body energy. They avoid an overloading of your kidneys by nullifying urinary wastes in your blood before they reach your kidneys. Being very low in salt and fat and having no cholesterol, they spare your heart. Since they are absorbed slowly, but "stick to your ribs," they save your pancreas from overwork. Bananas even have a high content of vitamin C. Their thick skins, of course, protect their pulp from sprays and insecticides. They are still comparatively inexpensive and are easy to handle and prepare. Born and raised until seventeen in a banana haven like Panama, I have always eaten them and continue doing so in the United States.

Bananas also mix with anything. For lunch, eat grapes first, for instance, then finish the lunch with bananas—or the heavier food. For the last few years, I have eaten the grapes and bananas together to let the banana absorb much of the residues of the sprays on the skins of the grapes. On principle, however, eat the heavier food last or just before the beverage. Otherwise, you will tend to get gas. Please don't consider these "wise eating" precautions fussy. I have tested them on myself for half a century, and my health is the envy of people everywhere. Let others deride you for taking intelligent care of your health. When you get sick, these people are the first ones to call you a hypochondriac or to snarl that you are "getting old." When you are ill, you alone suffer from your pains and discomforts. Nobody else suffers from them for you, no matter how much they sympathize with you, so ignore them and stay healthy.

MORE FOODS FOR LASTING POWER

Soybeans are another fine food to tone up your arms (or to tone up your whole body, for what tones up one part of it, tones up all of it). They are an excellent source of protein. If you are a man, they are an excellent synthesizer of semen, because the protein in your semen is qualitatively the same as that of your blood. Its amino acid content (the building blocks of your protein) is even higher than in meat or eggs, and sometimes is *much higher*. And the proportions of different amino acids is ideally balanced. Methionine, the lipotropic (fat-absorbing) amino acid which is low in vegetables, is most abundant in soybeans. Soybeans, in fact, contain almost 10 times as much calcium as meat, and about twice as much as eggs. They even contain more iron than meat, and meat contains the recommended standard amount necessary to relieve anemia.

Eggs surpass both meat and soybeans in vitamin A, a most necessary vitamin for your skin. Egg yolk is packed with it. Soybeans, however, contain far more vitamin B than meat, although meat is a rather good source of it. Do not substitute nutritionless starchy foods, like noodles, spaghetti and macaroni for meat. Some leading marathon runners fill up with such foods to last them through arduous races. Dates would "stay" with them just as well and nourish them besides.

FOODS FOR BEAUTIFUL (OR POWERFUL) ARMS

To acquire firm, trim, shapely arms (or powerful ones if you want that kind) you need all the nutriments you can get from your vegetables. To achieve this, never peel your vegetables before cooking them (that is, the comparatively few which are all right to cook). Their skins, it is true, are thickly coated with insecticides—unless you can afford to buy all your food from organic sources. But their skins are packed with vitamins and minerals. I prefer to scrub the hard ones with a strong brush and soap, and rinse them thoroughly. Cook vegetables (when you do) as briefly as possible, and in a very small amount of water. Don't make them too tender, or you will destroy their fiber and roughage, as well as their vitamins. (Boiling the potato is a good example). Don't eat the vegetables when they are still hard to chew. Even if you would extract more vitamins from them if left uncooked, they would wear down the enamel of your teeth. As I stated before, whenever you chew a resistant food for long, don't let the saliva in your mouth turn warm from the friction of mastication. Cool your saliva repeatedly with sips of cool milk, or the heat will erode your enamel faster. Better yet, grate such food, rather than depending upon your teeth to chew it down to digestible size.

Never soak your fresh food even if you retain and drink the water in which you cook a vegetable. Its vitamins have been heated out of it and partially exposed to air, and air destroys vitamins. Soak dried fruit like figs, prunes, raisins and pears to restore the water they lost during dehydration, as well as to soften them and save your enamel when you chew them. Soften them in tightly-shut jars, just big enough to contain them and thereby minimize the volume of air they are exposed to. After you serve portions of them from the jar, shut the jar at once to retain all the saturated air possible in it and prevent further oxidation of the vitamins.

YOU CAN'T GET QUICK ENERGY FROM ANY FOOD

Ignore ads that urge you to eat candy for quick energy, ice cream for the milk in it and dried cereals for their vitamin B content. These products are full of sugar (white sugar, besides!) which robs your body of vitamin B, while the processing of the cereals has robbed them of nutritional value.

Even the energy set free in your own body comes mainly from the oxidation of carbohydrates, which is executed in step-by-step chemical reactions. Enzymes (and coenzymes) trigger these chemical reactions within your cells and make the energy available *gradually*, or no faster than your body can utilize it. If the energy is released all at once, as it does after you eat white sugar with is "quick energy," you suddenly burst with energy as the sugar floods your blood, but soon collapse from fatigue as the sugar vanishes. When you feed yourself like that, you will exercise your arms very little, for you are soon too weary to be active or to exercise.

THE SLIMMING SECRET OF YOUR SPECIFIC BODY WARMTH

Whenever you eat, your metabolism increases markedly, and your body liberates about 300 calories of extra heat. This extra heat has *nothing* to do with the amount of calories you eat, and it is called the *specific dynamic action*. It is not created by the work of your alimentary canal in digesting your food. Eighty per cent of it, though, originates in your abdominal organs. That seems to associate it with the breakdown of the amino acids of the protein you eat and with their conversion into the waste product urea. This liberated heat also varies with all three organic foodstuffs. Proteins release 30 percent of the calories found in foodstuffs, carbohydrates release 6 percent and the fats release 4 percent. A mixed diet releases about 10 percent. This extra heat, it should be noted, cannot be used by your muscles and glands to perform their work for your activity, exercise, physical power, endurance, stamina and so forth. But it is valuable in a cold environment, where it can warm you up. It helps to keep your arms (and your body and waist) firm and trim because it lessens your appetite for more food to keep warm. Proteins, for that reason, are valuable foodstuffs in cold weather.

When you are undernourished, however, (such as, when you fast, skip breakfast or eat junk food) your body requires *more* calories to stay warm and energetic and extracts *more* heat (more specific dynamic action) out of everything you eat. But when you are overweight your body requires *less* calories to stay warm and energetic, and extracts *less* heat from everything you eat. Your body, to conclude, possesses the varying faculty to extract either *more* heat or *less* heat, from your food than your food normally provides. That explains why your basal metabolic rate is reduced and your body temperature is lowered when you are overweight. Conversely when you fast, your basal metabolic rate is *increased* and your body temperature is *raised*.

Here is the slimming secret of your specific body warmth.

1. Keep your body feeling *extra* warm when you eat, in order to absorb *more* heat from your food and thereby *reduce* your appetite.
2. Increase your feeling of warmth with the Triple Tonic Secret (Illus. 17) so that you *feel* like eating less. You won't have to *try* to eat less; you just won't feel as hungry as you did.

How Bertha A. Had to Wear Long Sleeves to "Keep the Men Off"

For years, Bertha A. had been ashamed of her arms. "They are so plump in the back," she moaned. "Like a work-horse! I bet that's why my boyfriend stopped calling me up!"

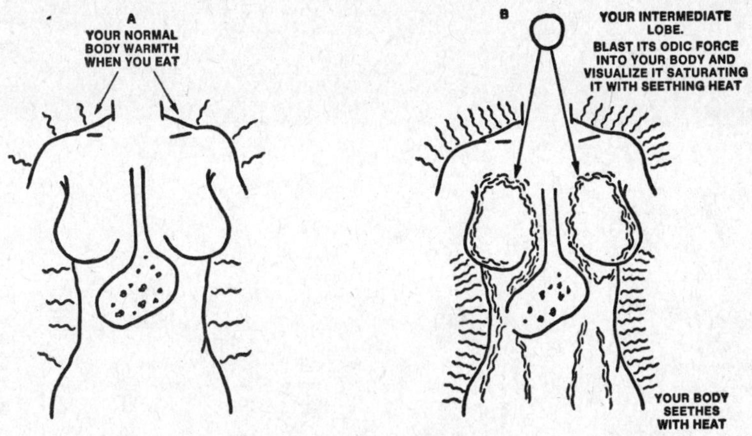

Illustration 17

Bertha's body and waist had gained weight, too, although not that obviously. With the *Yogatronic Diet*, her waist and body trimmed first, but her arms soon followed. In a few weeks, they became firm and took fifteen years off her apparent age. Indeed, they looked so sylph-like that she was compelled to wear long sleeves to discourage the many men who tried to stroke them when they associated with her. After her boy-friend caught one look at them, he pursued her relentlessly. With the slimming secret of her specific body warmth, Berthe melted off, in about five weeks, her remaining 14 lbs. of excess weight.

How Victor B. "Out-Skilled" His Rivals and Moved in for a Big Raise

For some time Victor B. felt as if he was "no more than average." He was astonished when I assured him that he would feel invincible once he had strong firm arms. In order to feel unconquerable with flabby arms, I told him, he needed an abnormal amount of self-assurance. With firm fatless arms, he would worry little that he was shorter, less broad-shouldered, less educated, and had a smaller vocabulary than his rivals.

The *Yogatronic Diet* trimmed down his arms in a few weeks, and he increased his activities with a vengeance. He "out-skilled" his rivals and moved in for a big raise.

18

Restore Body Agility—Through Yogatronics

YOUR MOST VALUABLE FOOD FOR BODY AGILITY

Without body agility you won't gain enough from a trim body and a small waist. You will have trouble retaining them without dieting because your muscles will soften and their cells will irreversibly turn into fat. Body agility, however, requires protein because it breaks down a part of your muscles through its exertion and rebuilds it with stronger cells.

But it can't utilize just any protein. Eight amino acids are essential to the rebuilding protein your muscles need to repair themselves. Whole corn is low in one, wheat gluten is low in three and gelatin is deficient in six. Animal proteins (except for gelatin) contain them all. Yeast, corn germ, wheat germ and soybeans are equal to animal protein. Muscle composes 49 percent of your body weight. Half of your metabolic, chemical and physical activities occur in your muscles, *even during rest.* That's why you *cannot* ignore your muscles if you want a youthful, trim body and a small waist. When your muscles contract or work, however, they use up fully *three-quarters* of your total metabolism. That's another reason why I oppose exercising too soon after your meals. Your body can't digest your food and feed your active muscles at the same time without straining your heart and giving you indigestion.

Proteins are the most complex and your most important foods, because they are the only ones that can build your tissues. Without the right amount of them regularly in your system, it is not easy to acquire an agile figure. Egg white is nearly all protein. Egg yolk, lean meat, fowl, fish, cheese, nuts, legumes and some cereals are other good sources of it.

HOW TO EXTRACT THE UTMOST FROM YOUR MOST VALUABLE VITALITY FOOD

The proteins you eat should be digested easily enough, so your muscles can utilize them more completely. That's why it is better to eat meat or other protein with a proteolytic (protein-breaking) enzyme-containing food, like pineapple or papaya. If you are a body builder looking for giant muscles, your muscles will grow faster after strenuous exertion if you eat these foods. If you want to lose weight, you must absorb protein faster and consume less fat. But I oppose your eating too much protein to build up or reduce, whether in natural food or in food concentrates. It produces too much pyruvic acid. You will excrete it as yellow urine (xanthurenic acid), which may be another cause of cystitis (inflammation of your bladder) if continued for a long time.

You should also extract the utmost value from your proteins. Proteins, for one thing, are not as stable as you presume. You can't abuse them before you eat them. When heated, shaken or subjected to certain physical forces, as well as to acids and alkalies, the insides of their molecules rearrange themselves and "denatures" them. Denaturing renders the protein far less soluble. When egg white (a protein) is boiled, for example, it is coagulated. Hence, don't eat your proteins with acid fruits or overheat them.

YOUR BODY AND THE HUGE MOLECULES OF PROTEIN YOU EAT

During your digestion the huge molecules of the proteins you eat are broken down irregularly by your stomach acids and enzymes. As your digestion continues it converts the protein into simpler and simpler substances. Proteins in legumes (beans and so forth) and in various cereals dissolve in water. When heated to about 75° C. (167° F.) they coagulate. Proteins, like liver and thymus gland, are rich in arginine, the sperm-producing amino acid. The mucins in your saliva, in your digestive "mucus," in the fluids within your eyes and joints and in the lining of your stomach, are proteins. They are slippery and have lubricating value for the passage of your food through you, for the accomodation of your lens and for the movements of your joints. They are not digested by the enzymes of your alimentary canal. Their presence in the slimy secretions of your stomach, intestines, eyes and joints protects these parts of the body.

How to Protect the Valuable Protein You Eat

When you eat proteins with fruit or other foods that are sprayed with the poisons of heavy metals (mercury, silver and lead), those metals combine with the proteins and precipitate them. The proteins, however, do not save you from these poisons unless you remove their precipitates with the heavy metals, by vomiting or by a stomach tube. But that would prevent their being digested and stop the heavy metals combined with them from being liberated again and absorbed completely by your tissues. The roughage of raw food helps to avert that catastrophe by absorbing the heavy metals before they combine with the protein and excreting them through your rectum. It considerably limits the amount of sprays and insecticides of heavy metals which would combine with the proteins you eat.

Certain acids also precipitate protein. That's why, as stated before, it is not wise to eat acid fruits, like oranges and grapefuit, with meat. But pineapple, because of its proteolytic enzyme bromelin, breaks down your protein for digestion. Don't eat hard-boiled eggs, even though they are on the menu of many leading health diets. Their coagulated whites will not dissolve in dilute acid (that of your stomach), or in dilute alkali (that of your intestines). That's what can happen to the protein of the lens of your eye when it is repeatedly exposed unprotected to sun rays. The light of the intense sun is strong enough to denature or rearrange the molecules of the straight chain molecules of your lens and cloud them. With added regular exposure the molecules become folded and result, as you grow older, into old-age cataract. That different arrangement between the molecules of a protein is responsible for the difference between straight, curly and fuzzy hair. Wood protein can be stretched, unfolded, and shrunk, indicating that the molecule is folded still more.

THE INBORN ABILITY OF YOUR CELLS TO RECOGNIZE ABNORMALITIES IN FOOD

Cells, certain researchers have found,[1] can recognize *abnormal* proteins and break them down rapidly into amino acids. This phenomenon occurs in bacteria, as well as in higher organisms. In hyperthyroidism (goiter) this breakdown is speeded up, especially in the cells of the muscles and the liver, and the victim loses weight and body proteins faster and stays thin. It is a dangerous type of thinness, however. This thinness is also the end result of muscular dystrophy. Now, *read the next paragraph slowly and carefully.*

The researchers showed that nearly all proteins are reformed and broken down many times within the life of a cell, although their speeds vary with your physiological condition. Besides, different proteins last for vastly different lengths of time before they are destroyed. Some are broken down after minutes, some after hours and some after days. Your body's control over these metabolic speeds is very important to biology and the clinic. These speeds appear to depend enormously upon the physiology and growth of the cell. In many important diseases, the proteins are broken down very quickly. Sickle-cell anemia is a prime example. Proteins with larger molecules, on the whole, are broken down faster than proteins with smaller molecules. So are the more acid proteins, and proteins combined with sugar, like the glycoproteins.

These researchers proved that your cells possess the astounding ability to "recognize" abnormal proteins, which is the firmest proof that you yourself *can* control your cells and extract the utmost nutriment out of proteins with the Triple Tonic Secret. With it, you can restore your body agility much faster than otherwise, and you can do so without food concentrates. Your cells aren't robot tissue that fatten or thin you by what you eat alone. They are independent personalities that pick and choose. With the Triple Tonic Secret you can direct them to pick and choose more masterfully, filling you with still more agility. You can then acquire a thinner body and a small waist much faster and more permanently. Here is that Triple Tonic Secret. (Illus. 18).

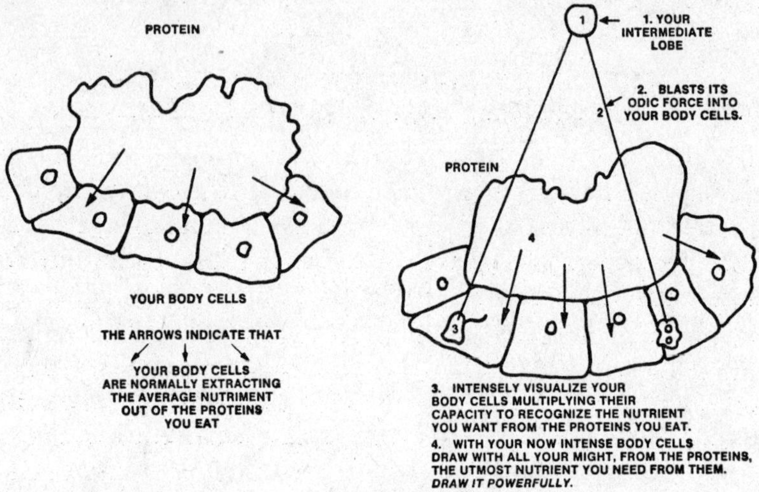

Illustration 18

THE FOOD YOUR BODY CANNOT SYNTHESIZE

Your tissues cannot synthesize protein as they can certain vitamins. You eat either animal or vegetable protein, digest them to the amino acids of which they are composed, absorb them and form your tissues from them. Certain amino acids are indispensable and essential to maintain your health, your trim body and your small waist. A lack of the amino acids tryptophan, histidine, or phenylalanine, for example, can cause cataract, as well as defects in the teeth, baldness, a decreased amount of red blood corpuscles, anemia, atrophy and defects of the sex organs.

You can't make up for the missing amino acids with beef extracts. They don't have the "strength of the beef," because the muscle tissue has been hashed, repeatedly extracted with hot water, filtered and concentrated. All that is left are small quantities of carbohydrate, amino acids and peptides. Clear boullion, too, has little nutritive value. Heat also alters the nutrition of protein. The proteins of egg white and navy beans are more nourishing when cooked. (but only, I insist, when cooked a little, such as by poaching eggs). Soybeans are improved by heat because they contain a toxin, soyin, which is inactivated and detoxicated when cooked. They also contain an inhibitor of the proteolytic enzyme trypsin, and heat destroys it. You can't eat soybeans with meat, otherwise, or the meat won't digest. That's also why toasted and "puffed" cereals should be avoided.

A STILL GREATER THREAT THAN OXALIC ACID

Protein, like sugar, supplies energy to your body, because its carbon chains form carbohydrate (sugar). That's why you can get fat by eating too much protein: the excess protein will turn to sugar.

To get more protein, don't overeat nuts, legumes and the *outer* layers of cereal grains. Not only will they fatten you, but they contain too much phytic acid. That's another reason why I don't recommend wheat germ oil. The phosphorus in these foods occurs as phytic acid. Like oxalic acid, phytic acid may combine with part of the calcium, magnesium and iron in you and sweep them out of you unabsorbed.[2] Indeed, oxalic acid seems to be less of a threat, because, according to researchers, "Relatively few foods have sufficient oxalic acid to deprive you of a significant amount of calcium and magnesium from either themselves or from some other source. . . . Peanuts, pecans and wheat germ contain moderate amounts of oxalic acid. Carrots, collards, kale, leeks, okra, parsnips, potatoes and sweet potatoes contain smaller quantities of it. The total amount of magnesium present in these foods is probably more than enough to combine with all the oxalic acid in them, and is therefore enough to leave the calcium in them practically undisturbed."

THE WISE WAY TO DECIDE WHAT FOOD TO EAT

At the time I competed with the young body builders of half my age and finished as a finalist against the future Mr. Universe, I warned them all against taking high protein body-building food concentrates to reduce body fat and build up fantastic muscles. I published this warning in *Solar Diet.* Few believed me.

Again I was far ahead of my time. Twenty-five years later, my warning came tragically true, and the FTC has cautioned against using liquid protein products to reduce. Yet I myself, at that comparatively late body-builder competition age, developed fantastic muscles in a few weeks with natural foods! Suppose I had taken body building pills like anabolic steroids, as so many do today! But health, to repeat, was always my main objective!

Here is another reason why I insist so much on natural food instead of extracts and concentrates, even if it is vastly devitalized in the big polluted cities. Bahrs and Wulzen discovered a relatively new fat-soluble vitamin, the "anti-stiffness factor." Without it your muscles atrophy and become streaked with unhealthy calcium deposits. These even extend under your skin and bring you an "aged" look. They extend into your joints and elsewhere in your body plaguing you with arthritis. A highly recommended food concentrate, like cod-liver oil, *accelerates* and *intensifies* the condition. So, if you take cod-liver oil for its widely praised vitamin content, you rob yourself of another necessary vitamin. The "anti-stiffness factor" vitamin is found in fresh kale or alfalfa, and in fresh cream. If you keep on taking fresh cream and avoid cod-liver oil, you will be supplied with your share of that necessary vitamin. I, like most nutritionists, don't advise you to take cod-liver oil, because of its high fat content. Too much will also over-stiffen your muscles.

On the other hand, when taken in skim milk after a meal with high-fiber foods, like a *Yogatronic* salid, cod-liver oil appears to be very beneficial for your skin, hair, nails, the lining mucous membranes of your eyes, mouth, alimentary canal, joints, blood vessels, heart and all other organs, without fattening you or disturbing your digestion. But take no more than the "normal" listed.

The best precaution, I believe, is not to overeat any particular natural food. But, don't condemn any outright and stop eating it altogether. Avoid food concentrates as much as possible. When they deprive you of a particular nutrient, they do so in a wholesale manner. Natural food is not concentrated and can deprive you of a particular nutrient only in a minor fashion and harm you very little.

THE ENERGY TRANSFER BOND FOR SUPER-POWER AND STUNNING TRIMNESS

To provide energy to your muscles when they contract you need the energy-rich phosphate phosphocreatinine bond. Meat,

meat gravies, meat soups and meat extracts contain it in profusion. I prefer to limit the source to meat and leave the extracts alone. When that phosphate bond breaks down, it releases heat and actively transfers its energy to another phosphate carrier, like adenosine triphosphate. Adenosine triphosphate contains *two* energy-rich phosphate bonds instead of one, each of which can transfer a tremendous amount of energy. The release of this "doubled" energy in your muscle fiber readies it for Herculean activity. The energy in the bond is released at two transfer points into the muscle, and each release is written PO_2H_2.

With the Triple Tonic Secret, you multiply the power of your muscles by renewing swiftly the energy of these transfer points. You do it when you take in new oxygen into your bloodstream. Do it now with The Triple Tonic Secret (Illus. 19).

Note: This is a most effective way to maintain ideal weight as you live longer (never say "get older"). As you live longer, you tend

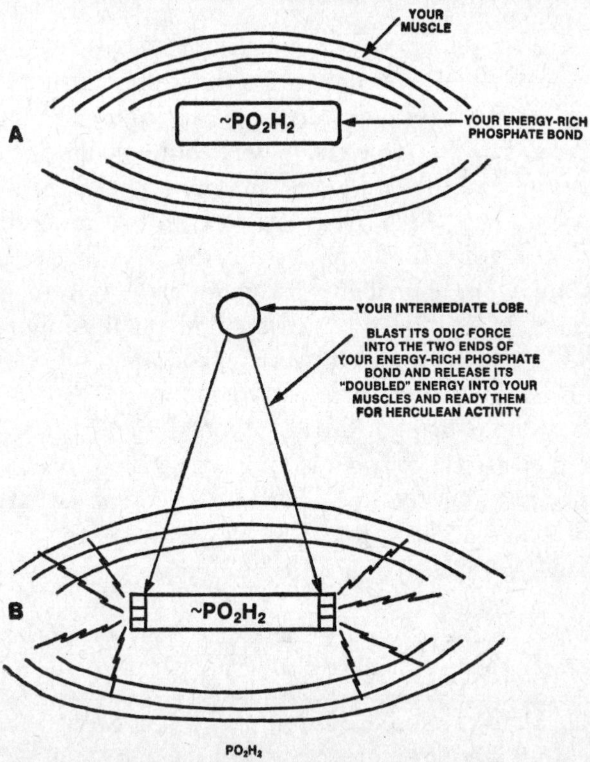

Illustration 19

to get heavier because your basal metabolic rate slows down. You will need less food, but you will retain the cultivated appetitie of youth, which has been transferred from your alimentary canal to your mind. (I insist, however, that if you have remained healthy, your gastric glands will also remain very active and your appetite will remain genuine). As you live longer, you tend to be less active and to exercise less. Less of the food you eat will be utilized by your body, and the unused food will be stored as fat. The healthy way to retain a youthful, trim body and a small waist is to continue eating your fill, but to exercise more. You should also stimulate your energy transfer points to their peaks just before you exercise to keep your muscles active longer. Exercise is of the utmost value. The whole world is realizing it 57 years after I did. Add to it the *Yogatronic Diet*, and it is the surest way to avoid a flabby figure and a jelly-like waist all your life—and to keep your mind, meanwhile, at its keenest. I have proved it in my own life.

How Hector N. Trimmed Down 68 Pounds and Felt Healthier Than He had Since He was a Youth

Hector N. had noticed, as he put on weight, that he tired more easily at work, was slower physically, and was less persuasive romantically. His bowels turned sluggish; he needed more sleep at night, and he lost the "energetic lift" he had in his prime.

With the *Yogatronic Diet* Hector's cells regained their inborn ability to recognize abnormalities in food. With the help of the Triple Tonic Secret, his cells extracted far more nutriment out of the proteins he ate and restored his body agility much faster. He had achieved it all without taking mega-vitamin pills, high protein or any other food concentrate. Gradually and healthily, over a period of about four months, he reduced his excess weight to his long-life ideal weight, and his waist practically disappeared. He could have lost it faster still, but the *Yogatronic Diet* reduces you with your health coming first. That's why Hector felt healthier than he had since he was a boy.

How Oona D. Hung on to Her Handsome Younger Husband Against Much Younger Competition

Oona D. had gained 31 pounds in her twenties and thirties and was losing her handsome, younger husband to a much younger slender woman. Oona tried different ways to control her weight, but usually suffered side effects. Also her weight returned whenever she eased up on a method in order to minimize its side effects.

I taught Oona the safe *Yogatronic Diet*, the one way that has been shown by science to be *the most effective and safe way* to lose weight. Her weight slipped off as if by magic without her curbing her appetite or keeping track of her calories. In a few weeks, she looked so much trimmer and younger that her straying husband noticed her with renewed interest and became romantically aggressive. Oona won him back completely from her much younger rival.

REFERENCES

[1]G.B. Kolata, "Protein Degradation: Putting the Research Together," *Science*, Vol. 198, No. 4317, 11, November, 1977, © 1977, by the American Association for the Advancement of Science, pp. 596-98. Quoted by special permission from *Science* and the author. Includes material about Arthur Goldberg and his associates at Harvard University, *Science*, and other researchers, like Ann St. John, now at Rutgers University.

[2]"Composition of Foods. Raw, Processed, Prepared." *Agriculture Handbook No. 8.* Agricultural Research Service, United States Department of Agriculture, p. 166. Approved for Reprinting, 1975.

19

how to balance your depleted foods with yogatronics

THE URGENT PROBLEM OF YOUR EVERYDAY VITAMIN IMBALANCE

It is impossible to have a youthful body and a trim waist unless your vitamins are balanced. If you regularly consume foods that are short of vitamin A, you will simulataneously deprive yourself of B-vitamins, of vitamin C, and probably of vitamins E and K. You will be doomed to suffering from weak vision, slow tissue growth, nervousness, delayed healing and repair of your tissues and capillaries, hastened aging and slow blood clotting when you bleed (including internal hemorrhages). You will not be driven to be sufficiently active (much less to exercise) to maintain strong enough back muscles for a straight, healthy posture and a firm trim waist. Even your food might not help much, because there has been a tendency on farms to shift to crops with lower mineral requirements instead of replacing the minerals in the soil.

Besides, it is not easy to determine whether you need more of one vitamin than another. If your thyroid gland is overactive, for instance, you might need massive doses of vitamin A. It might not be overactive, however, and yet you might need considerably more—or less—vitamin A than you suspect, because normal thyroid glands vary in weight from eight to 50 grams.[1] When you exercise violently, your body's need for vitamin B increases greatly for you lose much of it in perspiration. In active physical work your calorie requirements may be intensified by 80 percent or more, as compared to that of a sedentary worker. Without adequate daily vitamins and calories, however, you won't balance your diet. You will overeat to make up for them, lose your trimness and fatten your waist.

Balancing Your Vitamin Dosages Safely

Vitamin C protects your adrenal gland, which stores a comparatively high percentage of it. Your liver needs vitamins to change your food fats to body fats. It needs such vitamins as choline, inositol, vitamin B_{12} and all B-vitamins, as well as other food substances like lecithin and protein. Many B-vitamins and vitamin C help you from being poisoned by the chemicals in your food, and they are used up in the process. Vitamin B helps counteract alcohol, radiation sickness (you are subjected to radiation all day long), and cirrhosis of the liver. Vitamin C helps prevent the hardening of your arteries. Vitamin E helps protect you from blood clots and conserve oxygen in your bloodstream, thereby increasing your endurance and preventing you from tiring easily from activity or exercise. It also serves to discourage excessive scar tissue from forming and detracting from your appearance and to open up new pathways in your circulation when one of them is blocked by clots or hardened arteries.

To play safe, you are tempted to gulp large doses of different vitamins. But vitamins A and D are dissolved and deposited in your body fat and stored in your body. When you take massive doses of them for an extended period, you can create serious imbalances in the other vitamins, just as you can create a shortage of them when you take too little vitamin A. Cases of vitamin A poisoning have been reported.

If you take a moderate amount of vitamin A through its best concentrated sources (as from fish liver oil) your stomach and liver might not accept them. That's why I lean to natural sources like fish livers, eggs, liver, apricots, carrots, collards, beef liver, sweet potatoes and watercress. Vitamin A also occurs in dandelion greens, mustard greens, turnip greens and butter.

Note: Carotene forms vitamin A in your body. The vitamin appears in foods that are yellow or green. Some of these sources, however, like liver and turnip greens, are no longer desirable because they hold considerable added poisons. The other sources listed are less poisonous.

Many Common Drugs Destroy the Vitamins in You

A great number of the drugs people take destroy the vitamins in their bodies, even common drugs like aspirin or nicotine smoking. Estrogen, which is given to women during menopause and for birth control, produces a deficiency of thiamin and riboflavin, two major B-vitamins. Penicillin and chloromycetin destroy niacin. Streptomycin and the sulfa drugs eliminate folic acid, another B-vitamin. Arsenic (which is used widely on fruits and vegetables, except on organically grown produce) and sulfa compounds ruin para-amino benzoic acid, another B-vitamin, which is claimed to discourage the graying of hair. (I myself have eaten arsenic-sprayed fruits and vegetables for three-quarters of my life, nonetheless, and my hair shows hardly any gray). Penicilliamine (another drug) obliterates the B-vitamins and choline. Inositol, another B-vitamin, is blotted out by an insecticide. Biotin, still another B-vitamin, is annihilated by sulfa drugs and avidin, which occurs in the raw whites of eggs. Vitamin C is finished by sleeping pills, penicillin, nicotine in tobacco, and tannic acid in tea. Even raw fish (including shellfish and raw oysters) demolish thiamin (vitamin B_1). Medicines like quinine, given for malaria (of which I myself was fed gigantic doses during my long confinement for that disease in the Canal Zone hospital during my senior year in high school), and sulfa drugs slaughter vitamin B_{12}, the blood builder.

Even a laxative, like mineral oil, exterminates the fat-soluble vitamins: A, D, E and K. So do bleaching agents used in white flour, which leave little of its vitamins behind. Dicoumarol and the sulfa drugs devastate vitamin K.

Vitamins Against Vitamins

The vitamins themselves, in fact, liquidate each other, for they do not work alone in the body. They even work in combination with minerals. Meats (because of the sulfites added to them) and sulfured dried fruits (figs, prunes, pears, etc.) also nullify vitamins. Drugs containing toxic metals like lead, mercury, bismuth and arsenic kill vitamins. So do solvents, astringents, other laxatives beside mineral oil, alcohol, morphine, narcotics and pain killers. You already know about the large amount of each vitamin lost (even in organically grown food) following the picking: in the storing, transportation, exposure to air, light and changing temperatures, washing before consuming, preparing for the table (even from the grating and shredding, when not cooked), as well as during mastication and slow digestion, such as when you become active too soon after eating.

The Safe, Natural Way to Replace Those Lost Vitamins

As far as replacing those lost vitamins with synthetic vitamins, single vitamins, for one thing, are never found in natural foods, because vitamins do not work independently of each other. They *all work interdependently.* Vitamins, furthermore, are useless to the body—*except in the presence of minerals.* Vitamin B12, for example, contains two percent of the mineral cobalt in its structural formula. When soils lack this percentage of the mineral cobalt, no vitamin B12 forms in the plant. In humans, as another example, vitamin B1 does not act as such in the body. It has to be *converted,* first, into an enzyme, called carboxylase with magnesium acting as a catalyst. But, when your body is deficient of that percentage of magnesium, taking the vitamin B you lack will bring your body little or no benefit. Even if your food, in brief, happens to contain the right vitamins, unless it *also* contains the right proportions of minerals, the vitamins in it will bring you little benefit.

The best way, I believe, to replace these lost vitamins or minerals is with a natural food that is probably the least distorted by man, and which possesses a wealth of natural vitamins in the first place. My selection is a brown seaweed, like kelp, dulse, and the like. It contains iodine in the form of amino acids (in the identical form in which it occurs in your thyroid gland). Some varieties of seaweed contain as much vitamin B_{12} as is found in liver, which is the richest source. Vitamin E, which is poor in regular foodstuffs, is abundant in kelp. So is vitamin K. Dulse is said to have 300 times more iodine than whole wheat and 50 times the amount of iron.

An additional way not to lose more vitamins from your food is to boil your tap water in order to drive off the chlorine, and to let it cool before drinking. Chlorine uses up vitamin K.

How To Stay Young Vitamin-Wise

In a test on nearly 100 normal people, a difference of 10-fold was found between the amounts of vitamin C in their bloods. Your intestines synthesize many of the B vitamins, and your ability to synthesize your own will help you considerably to combat the shortages within you. Even sex makes a difference in vitamin synthesis, for women seem to have *less* choline (a fat removing vitamin B) than men. If you are a woman, it may explain why you are inclined to have more fat on your body than if you are a man, and probably why your blood pressure rises faster than a man's after your menopause. With the Triple Tonic Secret you can level off your body's greed for more of the vitamins it does *not* need, and stimulate it to synthesize more of those if *does* need. Here is the Triple Tonic Secret to achieve this desirable end and keep your body youthful and your waist small. (Illus. 20).

FATS, YOUR NECESSARY FOOD

Fats and oils, by weight, amount to between two and five percent of the average diet, but fats are necessary in your diet. They provide fat-soluble vitamins for your body, and they play an important role in your body's use of vitamins and minerals. But animal fats, like whole milk, butter, fat meats and lard, contain cholesterol, a leading cause of hardening of the arteries, strokes, heart disease, gallstones, and high blood pressure. Vegetable fats, in contrast, contain no cholesterol; they contain unsaturated fatty acids, instead. Animal fats are what contain saturated fatty acids.

The trouble is that *any kind of fat* is difficult to digest. Don't eat too much of any fat. Safflower oil, soybean oil, sunflower seed oil, corn oil, poppyseed oil and peanut oil are vegetable oils which either contain large amounts of *unsaturated* fatty acids or lecithin

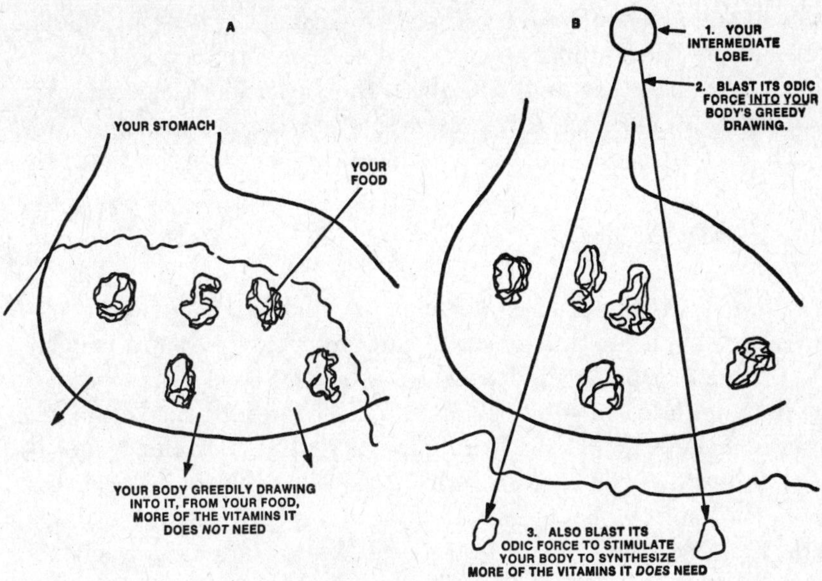

Illustration 20

(which is rich in *unsaturated* fatty acids) or both. They are better for you than butter, milk or prepared foods with white solid shortenings. Other foods abundant in unsaturated fatty acids are safflower, sesame and cottonseed.

The Natural Sources of Healthy Fat

Your body cannot synthesize certain fatty acids which are essential to your health, and has to depend for them on fatty foods. A large proportion of your fat is absorbed in the form of glyceride. That's why fibrous food (or roughage) can remove the cholesterol you eat as fat before you absorb it. Choline prevents excessive accumulations of fat in the liver. Here is a list of foods with choline, showing the units they contain of it: Lean meats contain 100 milligrams of choline per 100 grams of fresh meat; kidney, 200 to 300; brain, 350 to 450; liver, 450 to 600; fish muscle, 50-80; whole egg, 350 to 700; egg yolk, 1400 to 1700; whole wheat, 50 to 100; wheat germ, 350 to 400; oats, barley, rye, corn and rice, about 60 to 100 and yeast (brewer's dried) 240 to 360. Vegetables, as a group, contain little choline. Fruits contain even less. The edible fats you buy contain practically no choline. I still classify eggs as a valuable food. Their extraordinary amount of choline proves me to have been right about them all the time. They are full of lecithin, and choline has been found to be the active constituent of the lecithin molecule. Casein also saves livers from turning fatty.

How to Avoid Getting Fat When You Eat Fats

Your liver is your organ for metabolizing fats. When you consume too much fat and too little carbohydrate (fruit and vegetables), your liver is invaded with the excess fat from your food and accumulates fat. You get fat all over, including your heart, although vitamin E helps significantly to combat it. But, I prefer to get it from natural food such as more fruits and vegetables, and eat less fatty, cholesterol-forming foods. To avoid getting fat, avoid foods with saturated fats like lard, butter, bacon and margarine. Such fats are solid at room temperature. There is some fat, of course, in all vegetable substances such as nuts, avocados, sunflower seeds, peanuts, soybeans, whole grain, wheat germ, brown rice and walnuts. But vegetable fats don't put cholesterol in your body, which collects in your gall bladder, arteries and other places. In fact, they contribute a substance to your body which helps it use the cholesterol properly.

In animal fats there is fat in eggs. Eliminate pork products, hydrogenated shortening, baked goods, coconut oil, fats in dairy products and fatty meats. Eat cheese rarely, unless it is cottage cheese. Avoid all fried and processed foods. Don't eat much ice cream.

Natural fats (unsaturated) in their natural state, as in a seed, contain antioxidants (anti-oxidizing compounds) which prevent oxygen from turning the fats rancid. But the antioxidants are disintegrated in many of the processes to which you subject your cooking oils. Natural fats are most abundant in vegetable and cereal fats.

Another important reason for having a firm, rather than a fat, thin or flabby body is that muscle tissue is more compact than fat. It weighs more per cubic inch; it therefore occupies less space in your body than fat tissue and eases the load on your heart.

HOW TO GET THE BEST PROTEINS YOU NEED

If you abandon meat and depend for your complete proteins on vegetables, you will need a computer to figure out for every meal exactly how much of this-or-that food you need to build your protein. It is wiser to use seeds, nuts and legumes to make up for the protein you derive from "poisoned" meat and meat products, but don't abandon meat for them, for they are not complete proteins. In their order of value, the biological value of protein foods are: eggs, milk, meats, whole wheat, rolled oats, corn, white flour and beans. Tough fibrous meat is difficult to digest and has low biological value. *Very* fibrous meat may have little more biological value than white flour. If you engage in muscular work (or are very active), you need a diet rich in protein, particularly meat. Your body then retains its nitrogen (the basic element of protein) apparently to create muscle tissue.

Your bone marrow is intimately concerned with forming your blood, and you need meat for your bone marrow. But no one can estimate how much of it you need, because the range of the number of cells in the bone marrow of average people may differ by as much as 22-fold. You have to sense or equilibrate your sense of need for the amount of meat your body needs, as you do with vitamins (Illus. 20, page 219). You can then apply the same Triple Tonic Secret to help your appetite select the right amount of meat to eat at each meal.

THE VITAMIN THAT SLOWS DOWN YOUR AGING

A leading scientific team discovered new evidence that vitamin E slows down aging.[2] Vitamin E also reduces the waist and keeps the body trim.[3] But, as always, I prefer to get it in my food, rather than in concentrated preparations. It is found in high quantities in foods like eggs, leafy green vegetables, beans, grains. Vitamin E slows down the aging process by neutralizing the formation of your aging pigments in various tissues.

THE UNSUSPECTED FOOD THAT HELPS YOUR THYROID KEEP YOU YOUTHFUL AND TRIM

Your thyroid has a stimulating effect upon your total metabolism and thereby helps keep you trim and youthful. More than half of the iodine in your body is concentrated in your thyroid gland. Your thyroid stimulates your metabolism by releasing a hormone, thyroxine, which it breaks down to tri-iodo-thyronine, the peripheral thyroid hormone. Tri-iodo-thyronine has five times the physiological activity of thyroxine. Scientists[4] now find that the *sulfhydryl groups* of compounds have a "profound effect" in breaking down thyroxine to tri-iodo-thyronine.

Garlic is a sulhydryl group. It has the—SH group (the Sulfur-Hydrogen group) in its formula. It is therefore a most important food to help your thyroid keep you youthful and trim. So is seaweed, because it supplies your thyroid with the iodine it needs. That may be a decisive reason as to why I have kept my weight *right on the line* during my whole lifetime, while consuming gigantic meals.

How Clothilda I. Transformed Herself Practically into a True Beauty

Clothilda I. was "fading away," and her followers were whispering. "How pretty she must have been twenty years ago!" was their typical remark to each other. Clothilda sensed it and became frantic about her career. She had gone to several spas, she said, but they had not done enough for her.

After a brief talk with her, I decided that her body had not remained vitamin-wise. Although she had taken her food supplements, her body had greedily absorbed the vitamins it already had enough of, but had not absorbed enough of thouse it lacked.

The *Yogatronic Diet* and the Triple Tonic Secret promptly took her in hand. Even without taking food supplements, Clothilda's body soon lost its greed for the vitamins it had enough of, and synthesized those it lacked. The effects were phenomenal. In but a few weeks, she normalized herself from a "faded woman" into a true beauty. Her followers flocked around her again.

REFERENCES

[1]Arthur Grollman, *Essentials of Endocrinology.* (J. P. Lippincott, Co. Phildelphia, Pa., 2nd ed., 1947)

[2]*National Enquirer*, August 1976.

[3]A study at the University of Puget Sound, Tacoma, Wash. Researcher Dr. Jeffrey S. Bland, an associate professor of chemistry, on 24 student volunteers.

[4]*Science*, Feb. 24, 1978. Vol. 199. No. 4331.

20

the quick and easy yogatronic diet program: the science-proven key to permanent ideal weight, a trim body and long life

HOW SCIENCE SUPPORTS THE YOGATRONIC DIET ALL THE WAY

The *Yogatronic Diet* is not a theoretical or experimental diet which an individual professional healer or two has experimented with on a long list of patients over a limited period of time. It is a diet which I practiced on myself and hundreds of people for nearly 60 years. After perfecting it for nearly 30 years, I had it published in *Solar Diet*. Six years later, Dr. Lester Breslow, Dean of the School of Public Health of the University of California, and his colleagues, started keeping a close record on a population of 7,000 adults in California, and maintained it for *seventeen* years.

In the meantime, twelve years after *Solar Diet* was published, Dr. Ira Cain[1] and other researchers commenced a seven-year, million-dollar federally sponsored study of the health habits of another 7,000 Americans, which was funded by the National Center for Health Services and Development. These two large-scale investigations together consumed 24 years, involved 14,000 subjects, cost around $2,000,000, and were conducted by many of the most respected researchers in the field. Both groups independently discovered the very same health formulas for living a healthy long life which *I* had revealed and explained in detail all through *Solar Diet* more than 20 years before!

The Astounding Revelations of the Two Great Scientific Investigations

The University of California's 17-year investigation, headed by Dr. Breslow, announced their recommendations for good health to include the following requirements:

1. A good night's sleep (seven to eight hours).
2. Three square meals a day (no more, no less).
3. Regular exercise.
4. No smoking.
5. Drink moderately or not at all. (None at all, I insist).
6. Maintain reasonably good weight for height.
7. Eat breakfast almost every day. (*Every* day, I maintain).
8. Don't eat between meals.

The National Center for Health Services Research and Development's investigation, headed by Dr. Cain, announced their requirements as follows:

1. Eat regularly.
2. Don't snack between meals.
3. Eat breakfast every day.
4. Get between seven and nine hours sleep every night.
5. Keep your weight around normal. (Decade after decade, my own weight remains *absolutely* ideal, even to a fraction of a pound.)
6. Don't smoke.

7. Don't have more than two or three drinks a day. (I myself, of course, touch no liquor and recommend none at all.)
8. Exercise regularly.

THE UNBELIEVABLE STEPS BEYOND SCIENCE

The *Yogatronic Diet* hits the mark *on every score*. It goes even further than the 17-year investigation by requiring a breakfast *every day*, instead of "almost every day." The seven-year investigation agreed with me completely on this point. My magic rules for living a healthy long life could not be more scientifically exact! And yet I discovered them *without* a laboratory, *without* one penny of financing, *without* one colleague to help me, and had come up with results *totally in opposition* to the scientific dictums of the time! I had originally revealed them long before science, and investigative science now finds them to be *totally accurate*.

You have to wait no longer to take advantage of the *Yogatronic Diet* now that you know how thoroughly science backs it up. Besides, science merely discloses the conclusions of its long studies. It did not develop the *details* of these magic rules, which I have throughout the *Yogatronic Diet*. In these last two chapters, I will direct you step-by-step on the simple way to follow the *Yogatronic Diet* throughout your day, for the rest of your life.

BEFORE THE YOGATRONIC BREAKFAST

Upon arising in the morning, take two glasses of warm water. *One* glass is not enough. Visualize it flowing all through you.

THE YOGATRONIC BREAKFAST

At the table, commence with a big salad bowl. It helps your bowels in the morning and reduces the amount of cereal you need to eat. This controls your weight easier and limits the amount of phytic acid you consume. Here is the salad. It should consist of *raw* vegetables without unhealthy seasonings, of leafy vegetables like lettuce, endive, watercress, escarole and of solid, bulky vegetables like carrots, beets, parsnips and celery (the green variety, not bleached). Use these or other vegetables, of course, when they are in season and affordable. A good number of them are always available. *Do not* masticate these solid vegetables, or they will grind down your teeth. Use a fine food shredder or grater. I have found that grating by hand is the most effective, but it takes up time, tires the arm and discolors the holding fingers to a degree, even if you wear cloth gloves. Of late I notice that very satisfactory and effective salad makers (*not* juicers) are on the market, selling for around $150. Investigate them for quietness and effectiveness in grinding very hard foods like carrots and beets, *without added liquid*. If they satisfy you *in your home*, you will have made a most valuable investment in health, in saving time and in the appearance of your hands.

DON'T try to soften these foods by cooking—no matter how little. Exceptions to this rule are vegetables like winter squash, string beans and possibly potatoes. These should be baked or boiled with as little water as possible.

Some vitamins are lost by storage in the refrigerator and by the necessary scrubbing with brush, mild soap and water before they are grated. Give them a thorough, but *quick* rinsing. Don't let them soak in the water, but be sure to rinse *all* the soap off them. Grate or slice your lettuce last, or you'll lose a substantial amount of its vitamin C. Head lettuce can be grated. Leaf lettuce can be held in a tight bunch and sliced. It must be made fine enough, or most of it will pass through you undigested. Put the prepared lettuce at the bottom of your salad bowl and the grated vegetables on top of it.

HOW TO GIVE YOUR SALAD A NICE BUT HEALTHY TASTE

Grate two medium-sized apples and spread this raw applesauce upon the salad. Top your salad with a large serving-spoonful of fish. I like sardines, mackerel, salmon or some such fish. You could even use leftover fowl from the night before.

Follow the salad with a dish of prunes, four or five, depending on size. Follow that with a side dish containing a tablespoon of raisins, a tablespoon of cooked, whole-grain cereal, a level handful of grated or ground walnuts, sesame seeds or some other non-fattening nut, and three softened dried figs, sliced fine. Raisin and fig juice will further soften the nuts. The fig seeds should be swallowed without chewing, to save the biting surfaces of your teeth from their sharp edges. Always buy sun-dried fruits, not sulphured. It is true that dried fruits contain sugar, but it is sugar in organic form.

Follow with one or two soft-poached or soft-boiled eggs. Finish off with a glass and a half or two of skim or two percent cream milk. You are now ready for a big day.

Note: You save time in the morning if you scrub your salad vegetables the night before. Scrub enough for breakfast and supper, divide them between two bags and store them in the lower area of your refrigerator. If a large beet is to be divided for the two meals, wait until morning to cut it and wrap the unused portion so it is not exposed to air. In winter, set the morning portion of the salad out of the refrigerator all night, or you will chill your stomach at breakfast and prevent your digesting enzymes from functioning.

WHAT TO EAT BETWEEN BREAKFAST AND LUNCH

Between breakfast and lunch, drink three or four glasses of water. Have a glass or two about 1-1/2 hours after breakfast. Have another glass or two, about 1 to 1-1/2 hours after that. Drink *nothing* for an hour before lunch. That is what I recommend to eliminate the unhealthy habit of eating between meals.

Remember, any snack between meals encourages an acid stomach. The stomach seems to secrete almost as much digestive juice to put away a small snack as a big meal. Eating between meals also encourages your gastric glands to overdevelop and starts you on the road to acidosis. To help avoid acidosis, be sure to work your gastric glands *only three times a day*. Many busy and overweight people have eliminated breakfast to get along on two meals a day by having what they call "brunch" (a combined breakfast-lunch). The *Yogatronic Diet* believes that two meals a day are too few and may seriously disorganize the body's functions, and thus lead to bad health. Between-meal snacks not only throw your system out of order and bring on acidosis, they also disrupt the regularity of your peristaltic wave. The same applies to fruit and vegetable juices. There is no such thing as a fruit juice that *does not* require digestion. In the stomach, the liquid is separated more completely from the small amount of solid matter lying in suspension in it—the solid matter which colors it and gives it its flavor and food strength. This solid matter has to be digested. Filtered water, in contrast, leaves very little solid matter in the stomach to be digested.

THE YOGATRONIC LUNCH

If you aren't big or hungry enough, you can eat much less of these foods if you wish. The *Yogatronic* lunch consists of two bananas, two pears (or the same quantity of some other fruit in season), about six ounces to a half-pound of grapes, *no* apples (they sharpen your teeth when bitten and chewed, incline you to drowze through the afternoon, and you already had apples for breakfast), a boiled potato, from three to 12 dates, depending upon how strenuously you work or exercise, and no beverage.

Fine foods for a big light lunch are fresh or unsweetened canned pineapple, a big slice of watermelon or a huge cluster of grapes. Pineapple carries much bulk and is full of natural, energizing sugar. Despite its acid taste, it will alkalize your system faster than most other natural foods. It flushes your visceral organs, helps to clean them out, and thereby shrinks your waist.

Drink no milk at lunch time, as it takes too long to digest. Take little water at meal time, since you can take water between meals. It dilutes your gastric juices, and such foods as meat require an acid media in the stomach for the enzymes that digest them to function. Maintain your lunch as a bridge between breakfast and supper. Don't make it either a big meal or a fast. When I attended college and graduate school in my teens, I ate heavy lunches and fell asleep in class in the afternoon. When I attended school in my forties I ate a big but *light* lunch and remained fully awake all day, even more so than my classmates, nearly all of whom were but half my age.

WHAT TO EAT BETWEEN LUNCH AND SUPPER

Since eating anything between meals, except plain water, harms your stomach, the regularity of your bowels, your general health and the trimness and youthfulness of your body and waist, eat nothing between lunch and supper. Drink a total of about two glasses of water, starting one hour after lunch, but no more, because you might keep getting up too frequently at night.

THE COMPOSITION OF YOUR SUPPER

Prepare the same basic salad you made for breakfast. But, instead of covering it with grated apples and fish, spread some tomato juice and sliced tomatoes and a serving of cooked beans over it.

It is not necessary to count the number of calories you consume every day. Eat enough light food first, to keep your stomach from becoming too acid from the heavy food, which should follow. That will prevent you from overloading yourself with the heavy food. Meat, as a heavy food, is comparatively easy to digest unless fried or cured, and it is a filling food. It can consist of steak, liver, kidney, lean beef, veal or other lean meats and fish. People who stuff themselves with too much meat are people who studiously avoid eating salads. Consuming a big salad bowl every breakfast and supper, before you eat the heavier foods, will limit the quantity of meat you eat and yet not starve you for protein. Forget how many calories you need or don't need to eat a day. Eat your food to enjoy it.

Two slices of whole wheat, rye, soy or oatmeal bread are all the bread you need all day. Eat them at supper time. Never eat nuts at supper time, except a thin layer of unadulterated peanut butter on your bread. Nuts take too long to digest for you to eat them so late in the day.

Finish your supper with 1-1/2 to two glasses of skim or two percent milk. Milk is a fine supper beverage because it stays with you.

WHAT ABOUT FOOD BETWEEN SUPPER AND BEDTIME

Limit yourself to no more than one glass of water between supper and bedtime. I have reduced mine to half a glass so I don't have to urinate more than once or twice at night. Don't let getting up at night to urinate terrify you. I have done so most of my life, and my kidneys are in A-1 condition. Don't let people embarrass you because you go to the "john" several times a day either. It keeps your kidneys flushed and in tip-top shape and your bowels softer and easier to move. Take care of your health and pity the ignorant scoffer.

THE YOGATRONIC RULES FOR MIXING FOODS

Rule 1. Limit yourself to no more than two or three different fruits at one meal. Fruits are "temperamental" foods. Avocados, however, mix with anything. So do apples, bananas and, with some people, pears.

Rule 2. Vegetables combine excellently with each other. You don't have to eat them separately.

Rule 3. Meat combines with fruits or vegetables. Combining meats, though, has been known to cause disturbance in sensitive stomachs. Since meat is acidic, it is wiser to combine it with an alkaline food, like vegetables, rather than with another acid food, which would increase its acidity. Always strive to alkalize your acidic foods.

Rule 4. Meat and potatoes, or bread and meat, *might* cause some acidosis if your whole meal is predominantly acid. For most people, however, there is no harm in eating meat with potatoes, or meat with bread.

Whenever a food combination disagrees with you, avoid it. However, make sure it is the combination, not your acid stomach that is responsible.

SCIENCE'S WARNING ABOUT ALCOHOL

A noted researcher, it was announced on radio, made a thorough experiment about the effects of alcohol on you if you exercise. He made these discoveries: Don't drink before you exercise. Alcohol prevents an increase in the oxygen in your blood, which you urgently need when you exercise, and your heart feels the pains of angina pectoris, which occur when the heart muscle labors without enough "pure" blood. The same caution applies if you drink after exercise, when your muscles are demanding more oxygen than usual.

REFERENCES

[1]Dr. Ira Cain, acting project director of the California Health Department's Human Population Laboratory, who is also a professor of sociology at George Washington University, *National Enquirer*, Feb. 1, 1977, p. 3.

21

the right foods and right habits – the yogatronic way to a miraculous new you

THE INSTINCTIVE AND NATURAL WAY TO EAT YOUR FOOD

Civilized man and the society he has created have brought unnatural refinements into the act of eating. When the animal eats, it does not count its chews, vary its eating speed or adopt a long list of good table manners which have little to do with proper digestion. There is nothing nutritionally wrong with the knife and fork, in not making a mess of table, in not smacking your lips or in not spitting out the bones like a "pig." When you eat, however, eating is the important thing. When you eat and think of your food and of its taste in your mouth, your digestive glands secrete fully. The power of the mind goes a long way toward encouraging everything you eat to do exactly what you hope it will for you. Let your mind aid your digestion at every step. Let it help direct the food you eat to doing its duty more easily. Your mind then lines up all the molecules of the food you are eating to point in exactly the same direction, like a magnetized substance, making it more obedient to your eating wishes. That's what the Triple Tonic Secret does for you. The best food in the world will not do miracles for you, unless your mind helps. When your mind helps, only God knows what miracles you can accomplish.

WHAT HAPPENS TO YOUR BODY WHEN YOU EAT AT BEDTIME

When you have already had three meals a day, bedtime feeding is overfeeding. Many people, including myself, have followed my instructions and eaten three square meals a day for years—and retain their ideal weights. Three square meals a day allows your body long, natural rests between feedings and lets your organs, your heart, your digestive system and your metabolism resume their normal operations. Such natural rests let your cheeks and the area under your eyes fill out again and they empty the splanchnic pool of blood in your abdomen and thereby reduce the girth of your waist. They let the blood return to your torso, back, arms and legs and restore their energies. Instead of swiftly tiring during activity or exercise, you get stronger and stronger until your next meal. Your mind becomes clearer, too.

Lying down immediately after a meal seems to cause acidosis in most people. A good walk after a meal is best. Otherwise, sit down (but don't slop over) in a comfortable chair, read and let your food digest. Slopping over in a chair after a meal compresses your stomach and can cause indigestion, but you shouldn't sit so straight after a meal that you exhaust your back. Eating at bedtime can give you an acid stomach and also constipate you, filling your system with toxins.

WHAT TO DO WITH YOUR BODY AFTER EACH MEAL

Never exercise immediately after a meal. After a light meal (consisting of fresh fruit or vegetables), don't exercise for about an hour and a half. After a heavy meal, don't exercise for three hours or more. Walking *is* exercise, but it is of limited in nature and makes use mostly of the feet and legs, not your area of digestion.

After eating, don't bend over, stoop down, jump or disturb the contents or your stomach in any way. Sit and walk straight, and let your digestion proceed undisturbed. Four-legged animals can do such things because they carry their digestive apparatus in a horizontal position, but man walks upright. All bending, stooping or twisting should be done before you eat, or after your stomach is empty. As little as one or two bends, after a heavy meal, can upset your stomach and fill you with gas. You don't have to stalk about after you eat as if encased in a straight jacket, but don't do anything that can bring on trouble. Just keep in mind what not to do after you eat and act accordingly. Soon, you will form the habit of not doing such things after you eat. You will feel so much better from observing these rules, that the pleasure and longevity they bring you will be worth more to you than all the money in the world. The late John D. Rockefeller, Sr., with all his wealth, lamented that he could not buy a new stomach. The man with a normal income, but with a good stomach, possesses property which no amount of money can buy. Money can be measured, but the wealth of good health is beyond measure. No transplanted organ can equal a normal, healthily functioning organ.

THE EFFECTS OF VIGOROUS ACTIVITY AFTER A MEAL

Never *run*, of course, after a meal. Don't even walk fast or climb stairs (unless you have to). Don't hold your child in your lap after you eat if you can help it, which lets him/her press against your stomach. Don't even pick up your child and carry him/her around if you can possibly help it. All of this contributes to indigestion. If you child is in misery, you *might* have to sacrifice your health, temporarily, for his/her benefit. Don't make it a practice, however, to upset your stomach unnecessarily. Train your children to consider your health, too.

Indigestion, you realize, turns your stomach too acid and can lead to diarrhea, with a loss of needed vitamins and minerals. It is followed by constipation, the retention of wastes in your colon, and the resulting discomfort and auto-intoxication. Your abdomen will balloon out and ruin your figure. If you suffer regularly from indigestion, you can end up with gastritis and, eventually, ulcers. None of these conditions will bless you with a small waist, even if they emaciate your body and carve your face into the contours of a skeleton's. They leave you looking from 10 to 20 years older than you are.

HOW TO EAT WISELY WHEN YOU TRAVEL

The Hunzas, the long-lived Caucasus people and the centenarians from Ecuador all spend their lives in one limited locality. The rhythm regularities which their lives form with their regular hours of eating, working and enjoying pleasure, as well as the harmony acquired between their bodies and that particular climate, contribute to their longevities. In the "advanced" civilization in which you live, such a lifestyle is impossible to follow. If you don't travel because of your occupation, you travel to visit relatives, for pleasure, to tour different locales, to escape insufferable weather and for numerous other reasons. Your rhythm regularity is frequently disturbed, which interferes with your wise eating.

The best you can do is to try to counteract the damage to your system with the *Yogatronic Diet*. Travel usually involves long hours of sitting, standing and waiting and involves abrupt changes in time which upset your regular routines. The long-lived people of the Shangri-las don't always fare well after long travel. Many die shortly after they return. Once your bowels become sluggish or unpredictable as a result of their broken rhythms or evacuate less wastes than they do regularly, your body accumulates poisons and becomes more acid.

If you drive, don't remain for hour upon hour behind the wheel. Plan stops where you can sprint or jog a little, to prevent your circulation from becoming too sluggish. Carry your own bottled water, so you won't have to drink water you don't like or aren't sure is safe.

THE SECRET OF LONGEVITY—SCIENCE'S PROBABLE GREATEST DISCOVERY OF THE AGES

Science has now discovered, experimentally, the "Fountain of Youth" and the sure way to a very ling life.[1] Many scientists believe that a dwindling immunity in man is responsible for such diseases as arthritis, diabetes, kidney diesase and an increased susceptibility to infection. The T-cells, a type of white cell in both man and animals, provides resistance to cancer, viruses, bacteria and fungi. But these cells fail with age, and both man and animal lose their resistance to diseases that can then kill them off.

Experiments[2] in mice show that the T-cells can be *rejuve-*

nated. They are the part of the immunity system that fizzles out with age, but which *can* be brought back to the intensity they had in young adulthood! A single injection of T-cells from younger animals increased the resistance to disease of older animals by an equivalent of 18 to 20 years in man. It is possible to collect T-cells from young adults and freeze them for 40 years. When the adult is old, the frozen cells can be warmed again and reinjected in order to bolster his wornout immunity system (or his resistance to disease).

Another promising way to rejuvenate the failing immunity system of man was found in a third experiment, in which mice were injected three times a week with a chemical called *mercapto* ethanol. This chemical increased the T-cell immunity in the older animals. But the large doses of the mercaptan proved poisonous, and the scientists started looking for *similar* chemicals which are safe.

THE FORTHCOMING MIRACLE DISCOVERY OF THE AGES

Oils of garlic and onions can be converted to mercaptans. The only hesitation the scientists had against using mercapto ethanol to increase the T-cell immunity of the older animals to that of the potency found in younger animals was that the large doses necessary were poisonous. The truth is that the mercapto ethanol which they injected was an isolated, concentrated drug.

The *similar*, but *safe*, chemicals they are seeking now to replace mercaptan will be equally difficult to find. It is much safer to use a mercaptan which is present in or naturally converted by a food. As I explained, I am sure it occurs in garlic. Garlic is not poisonous, as proven by the fact that too many of the longest living people in the world eat it daily. It has not poisoned me, and I have been eating it regularly since the age of 22. For thousands of years, it has been famous as a germ-killing food, which makes it a perfect food to bolster the immunity system.

If you are no longer a youth, it will be impossible for science to collect your young T-cells and inject them back in you when you are old. But, since science has found that a mercaptan *does* increase the T-cell immunity in older animals to that of younger ones and that such an immunity is what enables you to live long, I urge you to eat garlic regularly and "rejuvenate" your T-cells right now.

It is obvious to me that eating garlic and onions regularly since 22 has "rejuvenated" my T-cells constantly. That's why I look, and am, so young for my age, and have every scientific reason to declare that I will live to be at least 300 years old. The long-lived peoples in the garlic-eating areas of many "old countries" are proof that they have retained their youthful immunities against disease. Even though I have lived year after year in three of the most polluted metropolises in the world, my zero-hospital and zero-sickness record since the age of 25 attest to my immunity. It is never too late for you to start doing likewise, for science itself has found that the young T-cells injected into an old subject can "rejuvenate" his immune system and bring him "The Fountain of Youth."

SCIENCE HAS FOUND CERTAIN FOODS THAT MAKE YOU UP TO 25% SMARTER

Dr. Christian Gillin, a researcher and top official at the National Institute of Mental Health (NIMH), a government agency in Bethesda, Maryland, acting chief of the Unit on Sleep Studies at the Institute's Clinical Center, revealed that tests showed that giving people choline made them up to 25 percent smarter by improving their memory and ability to learn. The brain synthesizes acetylcholine from choline, he explained, and acetylcholine increases the thought circuits in the brain, believed to cause memory. Choline, he went on, was found in foods like egg yolks, wheat and fish. Since lecithin increased the body's choline level, he said, and thereby the amount of choline in the brain, he believed that giant doses of lecithin could do for the brain what choline did. Some of the foods that are very high in lecithin are eggs, salmon and ground beef, according to John Weihrauch, a research chemist with the U.S. Dept. of Agriculture.

For 24 years I have insisted on the value of eating eggs regularly, despite the warnings of science against it. I also insisted on the eating of fish and whole wheat products—all of which are high in choline and lecithin. But, I believe and will always believe in consuming the natural doses found in natural foods, for I prefer to invite no side effects. So, without even knowing that it improved the brain, those who followed my teachings were improving their brains *without even suspecting it*.

Geniuses have existed, and men and women have improved their minds through the ages without taking massive doses of lecithin, and in doing so, have avoided side effects.

THE REPORT OF THE SENATE SELECT COMMITTEE

A group of health experts gave testimony before the Senate Select Committee on nutrition and human needs and incorporated their views and opinions into a government document titled, "Dietary Goals for the United States." They are urging the President to crystalize them into a national policy. Americans, the report states, are eating less fruit, vegetables and grain products, while sugar and fat make up 60 percent of their total calories. Since the turn of the century, it continues, there has been an increase in heart disease, cancer, cerebrovascular disease, diabetes, hardening of the arteries and cirrhosis of the liver. Dr. D. Mark Hegsted of Harvard blames the diet for bringing on coronary artery disease, which causes nearly half of the deaths in America. The report adds that grains and legumes are better and cheaper sources of protein than meat, and also urges you to eat more poultry and fish. The Committee recommends that Congres provide funds for a nationwide education program, and that the latest starting date for the program should be five years from now.

I still urge meat as the perfect protein, because legumes and grains are incomplete proteins. It is a pleasure to be supported so fully by such a body as the Senate Select Committee. The *Yogatronic Diet* gives you the techniques enabling you to be trim and young all your life. Start applying it for magical results today!

A PARTING WORD

This book is the result of independent thinking and personal trial and observation which commenced at the incredibly young age of 10 and which has enabled me to make miracle discoveries in diet and healthy living from 1 to 57 years ahead of the most advanced discoveries of modern science. Parts of it were acquired from the knowledge passed on to me from my almost 200 year old Yogi, medical and dental ancestry in Asia and Latin America; from my studies in the professional fields of medicine, dentistry and chiropractic medicine; from my lifetime pursuit of physical culture, which includes boxing, weight-lifting, swimming and track; from my own invented natural exercises; from my lifetime of personal experience in diet under the stress of life; from the experience of hundreds of other people on two comtinents whom I have known and taught what I had learned; and from my secret psychic explorations.

Since I courageously followed my own conclusions instead of the scientific dogmas of my day, instead of waiting until science finally proved them in the laboratory, I am a whole lifetime ahead in health and longevity. Doctors of my age are finally jogging today, while I started 57 years ago. I predict that it will take science another 57 years to accept all the miracle discoveries in this book. But *you* can gain from them *right now* by putting them into practice—providing that you are normal and healthy. If you are not, see your professional healer first. Prepare to reverse old age, to regain the trim body and waist of your youth and to live much longer than you ever dreamed was possible, even if you live in a comparatively unhealthy environment. Let's go ahead together, and live together to a healthy 300 years of age.

REFERENCES

[1]Dr. Takahashi Makinodonan, director of the Geriatric Research Education and Clinical Center in Los Angeles. *Chicago Tribune*, Jan. 29, 1978.

appendix

THE HISTORY OF THE UNEQUALLED 110-YEAR STUDY ON NEARLY 10,000,000 PEOPLE WHICH FINDS THAT THE "IDEAL" OR "DESIRABLE" WEIGHT IS ASSOCIATED WITH THE "*LOWEST DEATH RATES* FOR A GIVEN HEIGHT."

Table 1

MAJOR MORTALITY INVESTIGATIONS OF BUILD AND BLOOD PRESSURE
by Association of Life Insurance Medical Directors of America and Society of Actuaries

BUILD				BLOOD PRESSURE			
Study	*No. of Persons Covered*	*Study Period*	*Maximum Follow-Up*	*Study*	*No. of Persons Covered*	*Study Period*	*Maximum Follow-Up*
Specialized Mortality Investigation 1903	Estimated over 100,000 men	1869-1899	30 years	Blood Pressure Study, 1925	560,000 men	1915-1924	10 years
Medico-Actuarial Mortality Investigation, 1918	750,000 men	1885-1908	23 years	Medical Impairment Study, 1929	25,000 men	1909-1928	20 years
Medical Impairment Study Supplement, 1931	370,000 men and women	1909-1928	20 years	Blood Pressure Study, 1938	1,300,000	1925-1938	13 years
Build and Blood Pressure Study, 1959	3,900,000 men and women	1935-1954	19 years	Build and Blood Pressure Study, 1959	3,900,000 men and women	1935-1954	19 years
Build and Blood Pressure Study, 1979	4,000,000 men and women	1954-1972	22 years	Build and Blood Pressure Study, 1979	4,000,000 men and women	1954-1972	22 years

SOURCE: Association of Life Insurance Medical Directors of America and the Society of Actuaries.

If you don't care how bony you look, just as long as you live the longest possible, you would have to trim down to the Optimal Weight.

I did so for 8 years, from 22 to 30. I did it by leaving out all meat from the *Yogatronic Diet.* I felt so light that I needed only four hours sleep a day and was tireless. But everybody felt sorry for me and thought I was wasting away. It is *not* a beauty weight. So I returned to the Ideal Weight and have apparently done as well healthwise—and look my most attractive besides.

The Optimal Weight is the weight of the marathon runner. It is not that of the matinee idol, of the beauty contest winner, of the sex symbol, of the teenage heart-throb, of the young-looking middle aged or elderly. Indeed, it is the weight of the one who looks prematurely old or convalescing from a serious illness or operation. No man who is 6-2 but weighs only 154 lbs., for example, has a physique that captivates the eye. Tables 2 and 3, for men and women, nonetheless, are important findings in the new Build and Blood Pressure study. You know how you can achieve it, if you wish, with the Yogatronic Diet, without fasting.

Table 2

MORTALITY EXPERIENCE FOR INSURED MEN AGED 40-69[1] AT OPTIMAL[2] AND AVERAGE WEIGHTS COMPARED TO STANDARD EXPERIENCE[3]

Study	MORTALITY EXPERIENCE BY HEIGHT AND WEIGHT RANGES											
	SHORT (5'3" — 5'6")				MEDIUM (5'7" — 5'10")				TALL (5'11" — 6'2")			
	Optimal Weight Range in Pounds	*Mortality at Optimal Weight*	*Average Weight in Pounds*	*Mortality at Average Weight*	*Optimal Weight Range in Pounds*	*Mortality at Optimal Weight*	*Average Weight in Pounds*	*Mortality at Average Weight*	*Optimal Weight Range in Pounds*	*Mortality at Optimal Weight*	*Average Weight in Pounds*	*Mortality at Average Weight*
1979 Build and Blood Pressure (Provisional data for 1954-1972)	150-159	99%	154	101%	155-164	97%	170	98%	165-174	91%	186	98%
1959 Build and Blood Pressure (Data for 1935-1954)	135-144	96%	150	97%	140-149	91%	167	98%	145-154	79%	185	93%

[1]*The age range of 40-69 has been singled out for illustration because this group tends to have particular problems with overweight.*

[2]*Optimal weight is the range of weights associated with the lowest mortality.*

[3]*Standard experience is measured at 100%; therefore, 105% means 5% higher than standard and 95% means 5% lower than standard.*

SOURCE: Ad Hoc Committee of the New Build and Blood Pressure Study, Association of Life Insurance Medical Directors of America and Society of Actuaries.

Table 3

MORTALITY EXPERIENCE FOR INSURED WOMEN AGED 40-69[1] AT OPTIMAL[2] AND AVERAGE WEIGHTS COMPARED TO STANDARD EXPERIENCE[3]

	MORTALITY EXPERIENCE BY HEIGHT AND WEIGHT RANGES											
	SHORT (4′11″ — 5′2″)				MEDIUM (5′3″ — 5′6″)				TALL (5′7″ — 5′10″)			
Study	*Optimal Weight Range in Pounds*	*Mortality at Optimal Weight*	*Average Weight in Pounds*	*Mortality at Average Weight*	*Optimal Weight Range in Pounds*	*Mortality at Optimal Weight*	*Average Weight in Pounds*	*Mortality at Average Weight*	*Optimal Weight Range in Pounds*	*Mortality at Optimal Weight*	*Average Weight in Pounds*	*Mortality at Average Weight*
1979 Build and Blood Pressure (Provisional data for 1954-1972)	115-124	90%	128	97%	125-134	94%	140	95%	140-149	92%	155	98%
1959 Build and Blood Pressure (Data for 1935-1954)	105-114	80%	130	95%	115-124	85%	144	96%	125-134	86%	160	107%

[1]*The age range of 40-69 has been singled out for illustration because this group tends to have particular problems with overweight.*

[2]*Optimal weight is the range of weights associated with the lowest mortality.*

[3]*Standard experience is measured at 100%; therefore, 105% means 5% higher than standard and 95% means 5% lower than standard.*

SOURCE: Ad Hoc Committee of the New Build and Blood Pressure Study, Association of Life Insurance Medical Directors of America and Society of Actuaries.

THE 5 WEIGHTS YOUR BODY CAN HAVE— AND WHAT EACH ONE BRINGS YOU

1. *Overweight.* Loss of beauty, agility, health, shorter life, early matronly look.
2. *Unnaturally Stimulated Muscle Size.* The overweight (whether muscle or fat) shortens your life. The gland stimulants taken endanger health. Unappealing in clothes.
3. *Average Weight.* Shortens life. In appearance you "look like everybody else." Do not stand out in clothes, in sport's attire, or in bathing suit. Waistline not distinctive.
4. *Optimal Weight.* Loss of beauty and the youthful look. In clothes look like "skin and bones." Chest and breast flat, neck stringy, arms shapeless, shoulders look weak, legs too thin. Life lengthened to the hilt, but look old very young.
5. *Ideal Weight.* Exhibits and retains beauty the longest. Excellent for long life and health. Retains the youth-look the longest. Waistline elegant. Eye-catching in any type of clothing. Looks most like a leader, a sex symbol, a professional man or woman, a model, a romantic lover.

I select the Ideal Weight as the most desirable weight of the five. Achieve it easily with the *Yogatronic Diet*, while eating "like a horse."